ANGUISH

MEDICINE IN SOCIETY SERIES
General Editors: Malcolm Johnson, Una Maclean and
Peter Sheldrake

ASPECTS OF ILLNESS
Robert Dingwall

MIRRORS AND MASKS
Anselm L. Strauss

STUDIES IN EVERYDAY MEDICAL LIFE
Michael Wadsworth and David Robinson

ANGUISH

A Case History of a Dying Trajectory

BY

ANSELM L. STRAUSS

AND

BARNEY G. GLASER

UNIVERSITY OF CALIFORNIA MEDICAL CENTER
SAN FRANCISCO, CALIFORNIA

MARTIN ROBERTSON

First published in the U.K. 1977 by
Martin Robertson & Company Ltd.
17 Quick Street, London N1 8HL

ISBN 0 85520 224 6

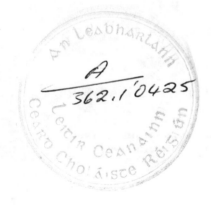

Printed in Great Britain by
Fletcher & Son Ltd, Norwich

CONTENTS

INTRODUCTION

The partnership of Barney Glaser and Anselm Strauss has been an especially productive one which has yielded an important product for sociology and another for those who plan and carry out care of the sick and dying. This volume, newly available to readers outside the USA, is important in both of these senses. It adds detail to the intricate sociological jigsaw which has been painted in *Status Passage* and *The Discovery of Grounded Theory*. It provides an insightful account of the much neglected issues in terminal care and treatment of people in death.

Although it can be read fruitfully alone, *Anguish* will be sought out by many sociologists and social psychologists for the contribution it makes to the literature on human social processes. The authors' earlier work has been characterised by an abiding concern with process and its relation to the temporal dimension of life. In carrying out their researches they have provided significant developments in methodology, the generation of theory from data and the extension of sociological concepts (such as career and biography) beyond their conventional boundaries. Here these strands are woven together in one case study.

In recent years the case study has gained some respectability in social science, having been previously overwhelmed by the numerical potency of the social survey. But despite the renewed emphasis on intensive small scale studies it is extremely rare for a single case to become the sole subject of a book. Indeed few authors would have the assurance and the courage to exemplify their work in this way. Nonetheless the story of Mrs Abel and the account of her trajectory towards death is moving, authentic, instructive and sociologically rewarding. It amplifies the theoretical propositions drawn out in *Awareness of Dying* and secures the case for analysing personal change as a permanent feature of human biographies, rather than treating it as a series of relatively scheduled life events.

Whilst observing the contrasting ways in which medical staff, nurses and Mrs Abel perceive her condition and what should be done about it, the reader is brought close in to a common and universal set of problems. There is nothing peculiarly American about this presentation of a terminal illness. It has all the problematic ingredients of Western medicine and the pre-death patient. The failure to tell the sick person the true state of their health, the personal and professional protectionism of staff, the ambivalence of staff to commit themselves to clear courses of action because of the unpredictability of the situation.

Glaser and Strauss's work on death and dying did much to bring the topic out into the social scientific open. Anthropologists have written extensively about death, but its systematic study in Western societies has been left largely to the medical profession. Yet, through their series of publications on the subject the authors have demonstrated the vital need for a non-medical perspective and indeed the many deficiencies of the medical management of terminal care. Nowhere is this made more plain than in *Anguish*.

For the student of careers, biographies and the interactions and negotiations which make up the fabric of status passage, this volume provides the closest account available of the research process itself. Fieldwork in this mode of enquiry remains very much a craft to be learned by bitter experience. In the unfolding of the drama of Mrs Abel's final weeks, she figures as the main actor, but woven into the story are the many other participants – not least the researchers and their problems and progressions.

So for a variety of reasons and for a number of different readerships this book makes a welcome appearance.

May 1977   *Malcolm Johnson*
                                                         University of Leeds

Barney Glaser and Anselm Strauss, *Status Passage*, Routledge and Kegan Paul, London, 1971.

Barney Glaser and Anselm Strauss, *The Discovery of Grounded Theory*, Weidenfeld and Nicolson, London, 1967.

Barney Glaser and Anselm Strauss, *Awareness of Dying*, Weidenfeld and Nicolson, London, 1965.

TO SHIRLEY AND SHIZU

CHAPTER I

THE CASE OF A LINGERING, DYING TRAJECTORY

This is the story of a lingering, dying trajectory—a long-term course of dying in a hospital. The shape of this trajectory had two major features: it was of long duration, and it moved slowly but steadily downward. When people die this way in America, most often they spend their last days, weeks, or even months in hospitals where an assessment of their condition is continually made. As this assessment varies staff members give them medical and nursing care —a hospital career—appropriate to each phase of the trajectory. In the instance of Mrs. Abel, a patient with cancer, whose decline exemplified lingering dying, she spent four months in the hospital during which her diagnosis took some weeks to make and to become generally known throughout the staff.

From a sociological perspective, the important thing about any medical diagnosis, whether correctly established or not, is that it involves two essential questions of definition. The first of these questions refers to "uncertainty of death," the second to "time of death." Even with a known terminal patient, "how fast will the patient die" must still be answered. Our concept of trajectory refers to *perceived* courses of dying, not, however well the fit, to the actual course.

Mrs. Abel's dying was perceived by the physician as certain and as occurring while still at the hospital, but his assessment of when was neither precise nor ever conveyed to the nursing staff. When the nurses finally realized that their patient was dying, they still did not dream she would die at the hospital because they conceived her death as temporaly far off. Later they were forced by developing circumstances to redefine her trajectory in terms of "will die here for certain" but for many weeks they were quite unsure as to how long that dying would take.

One main property of any lingering trajectory is its potential unpredictability, with regard to both the biological and human or psychological aspects of dying. The slow decline is fraught with hazard and opportunity. On the hazard side, the dying may take too long; the bodily deterioration may be unexpectedly painful or unpleasant; the patient may become terribly depressed when he understands that he is dying. On the other hand, slow decline may allow a person time to make his will, round off unfinished business and family affairs, and even permit a somewhat estranged couple to settle differences. Slow dying can permit staff members to participate in courageous or tranquil trajectories, but it can also involve them in stormy sessions and harassed days from family and patient. Mrs. Abel's dying vividly exemplifies the hazards of slow dying, with consequences for all concerned that can only be called negative.

In telling the story (in effect, a case history) of this lingering trajectory, we touch on sectors of at least four other stories. *First,* there is the "life story" of the patient. Something, but not all nor even a major part of her biography is woven into the case history. The most relevant part of her biography for our purposes is, of course, her lingering trajectory. *Second,* there is the story of how the hospital staff on a particular service reacted to, and interacted with their difficult patient during her slow decline on their terrain. *Third,* there is embedded in the case history the story of the two student nurses who, under the direction of Strauss, provided the bulk of the data about this trajectory: one did fieldwork which was focused on Mrs. Abel while the other provided special nursing care for her during her time on the service. Their combined story is one of two nurses coming to terms with their own reactions to death and to a most disagreeable patient. And *finally,* embedded in the case history also is the story of a final stage of a research project which had begun five years previously and was now rounding off with several publications.[1]

Before commenting further about these four subsidiary stories in our case history, it will help to explain how this case came to be followed and then written up. The research project alluded to above, consisted of intensive study of the interaction between terminal patients and several hospital staffs on a number of different types of hospital wards. The principle aim of the researchers was to gen-

[1]
Barney G. Glaser and Anselm L. Strauss, *Awareness of Dying,* (Chicago: Aldine Publishing Co., 1965); and Barney G. Glaser and Anselm L. Strauss, *Time For Dying,* (Chicago: Aldine Publishing Co., 1968); also our colleague, Jeanne Quint, had already worked out the framework for her monograph of student nurses, *The Nurse And The Dying Patient,* (New York: Macmillan Co., 1967).

erate simultaneously a substantive theory about dying in hospitals, grounded in the field data, while achieving relatively good verification of evidence through comparative fieldwork. This was accomplished well before encountering Mrs. Abel.

Once discovered, we decided to follow her course of dying, day by day, although her case added nothing essential to what we already know about lingering dying in hospitals. By this time, we had written one book and outlined another.[2] We were surprised by some events of this specific trajectory and certainly could not have predicted its outcome in detail, but we were never at loss for explanations as the case history evolved.

Why then did we bother to follow the case? It happened this way. Because of the previous study, Strauss became interested in another problem: how hospital staffs "manage" patients who are in pain. Mrs. Stephan Teale, a nurse who was studying for her masters degree in nursing, but also taking special work in field observation and interviewing, was given the task of doing fieldwork on several wards where patients were in pain. When first noticed, Mrs. Abel was only one of many patients discussed in the research student's fieldnotes. Eventually Mrs. Abel seemed such an informative case—she had become the patient on her ward with whom the staff was most preoccupied—that the student focused almost exclusively on how the staff was reacting to Mrs. Abel and she to them. Within a few weeks, the student and Strauss (who was following the evolving story through the student's reporting) suspected that Mrs. Abel would die in the hospital unless sent elsewhere to die.

Shortly after, the student researcher discovered on the ward another nursing student, Mrs. Shizu Fagerhaugh, who was taking work beyond her masters degree (post-masters). She had chosen as part of a class assignment to work with Mrs. Abel, giving her special nursing care every few days. She had chosen this patient because she suspected she was terminal and wished to nurse someone who was dying. At first the student researcher did not reveal to the student nurse, whom she knew, that she was studying this same patient. Until, some weeks later after she explained her own frequent visits to the ward, she regarded the student nurse as an especially important person to observe and interview.

After Mrs. Abel's death, the two women and Strauss spent three days reviewing events of the previous four months of her dying. The women reconstructed the salient events talking from their chronologi-

2
Ibid.

cal notes. The constructed case document then consists of their remarks, and Strauss' occasional queries, comments designed to clarify the events, and instructions about doing further interviewing to check out those details necessary to rounding out the story of the trajectory. One need not accept everything in the entire account as accurate, but by and large its internal consistency is sufficient to suggest a relatively accurate rendition of the unrolling course of events, both objective and in the eyes of beholders.

The interweaving of these four sub-stories with the story of the lingering trajectory yields a rich fabric and a highly detailed and complex history. Although there is only one main story, a burden is put upon the reader that he does not have to carry when reading conventional case histories. The unit (the story of a trajectory) on which we have focused requires a more complex case history than readers are accustomed to. However complicated is the story-line of the usual case history—usually a life history—still it tends to have one central focus and straight-forward plot. In contrast developing the trajectory requires our case history to shift back and forth from one sub-story to another. And seemingly out of chronological order, an episode may be mentioned which pertains to the history of the two student nurses, anticipating by a matter of weeks or months the chronology of Mrs. Abel's final days. Our case history also runs the danger of appearing repetitious in detail since episodes which figure in any one of the four sub-stories reappear eventually in all the others—so that, for example, an encounter between one of the student nurses and the head nurse becomes an event used to emphasize different points of some importance which is in each of the four separate sub-stories. We have attempted to reduce the repetitious quality of these narrations but some still exist. Readers need to be alert to the nuances of these repeated episodes, otherwise in tending to press on with the "main story" they may feel frustrated or wonder why the manuscript was not more severely edited.

If he can manage to suppress a natural inclination to get on with the story—remembering that a case history is after all not a novel nor need be merely an exciting, informative description—then the reader not only may find himself appreciating the sociological depth and richness of this kind of dying trajectory, but may find himself re-reading the case history with an eye to one or another of the four sub-stories. Some readers may be more interested in how hospital services function when confronted by such difficult patients as Mrs. Abel. Others may be more interested in a patient's reactions to her impending death. Nursing educators may be much interested in the student nurses' reactions as well as to how students versed in current nursing philosophy may still fail with this kind of patient.

Some readers, we would hope, would also wish to examine the qualities and functions of this case study in conjunction with earlier publications issuing from the same research project.

As the narrative of the case history appears here, it is divided into the following three chapters. In Chapter II, Mrs. Abel's death, and the immediate events leading up to it, are described. Chapter III covers the months when the staff was mainly focused on Mrs. Abel's pain. Chapter IV carries the story down through "last months, weeks and days" until death.

At the end of each chapter, Strauss and Glaser have added a theoretical commentary. These commentaries for Chapters II and IV are based on the substantive theory reported in their two earlier books on dying. The commentary about Chapter III is based on substantive theory developed both during the earlier research and on research done on "pain management" just before and after as well as during Mrs. Abel's last months at the hospital.

These theoretical commentaries differ in two essentials features from those which accompany most case histories. First, the theory which is applied to the case is *substantive* rather than the more generalized (or "formal" or "grand") type of theory which is more usually applied. Second, this substantive theory is *grounded* in research into the substantive areas within which the case falls. Our use of this substantive theory to the exclusion either of other highly general theories or ones drawn from distant sources—as is much more usual in case history commentary—is deliberate. It is meant to highlight and explicate the trajectory *rather* than any of the four substories. In the next section to this chapter, we briefly summarize our theories on dying, and locate Mrs. Abel's specific case within their generality.

DYING TRAJECTORIES, THE ORGANIZATION OF WORK AND EXPECTATIONS OF DYING

Before commencing the case history it is important to locate Mrs. Abel's own type of dying trajectory—lingering—within a general picture of types of dying trajectories as they relate to the temporal organizations of hospital work, the accountable features of terminal care, and the progressive change of the staff's expectations of dying.

Temporal Features of Terminal Care: While not entirely medical or technical, most writings about terminal care focus on the psychological or ethical aspects of behavior toward dying persons.[3] These emphases flow from generalized considerations of death as a philosophical problem, and the psychological and often ethical difficulties accompanying death and dying. Just as legitimately, however, the behavior of people toward the dying may be viewed as involving "work". This is just as true when a person dies at home as when he dies in the hospital. Usually during the course of his dying he is unable to fulfill all his physiological and psychological needs. He may need to be fed, bathed, taken to the toilet, given drugs, brought desired objects when too feeble to get them himself, and near the end of his life, even "cared for" totally. Whether the people who are in attendance on him enjoy or suffer these tasks, they are undeniably "work". Wealthier families sometimes hire private nurses to do all or some of this work. In the hospital, there is no question that terminal care, whether regarded distastefully or as satisfying, is viewed as work. Mrs. Abel required considerably physiological and psychological care which became progressively distasteful to the staff.

This work has important temporal features. For instance, there are prescribed schedules governing when the patient must be fed, bathed, turned in bed, given drugs. There are periodic moments when tests must be administered. There are crucial periods when the patient must be closely observed, or even when crucial treatments must be given or actions taken to prevent immediate deterioration—even immediate death. Since there is a division of labor, it must be temporally organized. For instance, the nurse must have the patient awake in time for the laboratory technician to administer tests, and the physician's visit must not coincide with the patient's bath or even perhaps the visiting hours of relatives. When the patient's illness grows worse, the pace and tempo of the staff's work shifts accordingly: meals may be skipped and tests less frequent, but the administration of drugs and the reading of vital signs may be more frequent. During all this work, any turnover among staff members, or their absence because of vacations or illnesses, must be managed through calculated organizational timing. This temporal management became more difficult and more liable to breaking down, as the nursing and medical staff progressively avoided Mrs. Abel because of her physical deterioration and incessant psychological demands upon the staff.

With rare exceptions, medical services always include a complement of recovering as well as dying patients. On quick dying wards, such as intensive care units, and on lingering wards, such as Mrs. Abel's cancer service, not all patients are expected to, or do, die. On

3
Bibliography in Robert Fulton (ed.), *Death and Identity*, (New York: John Wiley, 1965), pp. 397-415.

any given service, the temporal organization of work with dying patients is greatly influenced by the ratios of recovering and dying patients, and by the types of recovering patients. For instance on services for premature babies, most babies who do die do so within forty-eight hours of birth, but after that most are relatively safe. The "good premie" does not stay very long on the service, but moves along to the normal babies' service. Hence the pace and kind of work with a premature baby varies in accordance with the number of days since his birth, and when a baby begins to "turn bad" a few days after birth—usually unexpectedly—the pace and kind of work is much affected. On Mrs. Abel's ward nurses preferred to focus care and attention on recovering and less troublesome dying patients.

The temporal ordering of work on given services is also related to the predominant types of death in relation to normal types of recovery. As an example, we may look at intensive care units: some patients there may be expected to die quickly, if they are to die at all; others need close attention for several days because death is a touch-and-go matter; while others are not likely to die but do need temporary round-the-clock nursing. Most who will die here are either so heavily drugged as to be temporarily comatose or are actually past self-consciousness. Consequently, there is little need for nurses or physicians to converse with those patients, as there is on lingering wards, where we find Mrs. Abel. She continually wished to talk to nursing staff and her doctor no matter how pressed they were to keep working.

Each type of service tends to have a characteristic incidence of death, and speed of dying, which together affect the staff's organization of work. Thus, on emergency services, patients tend to die quickly (they are accident cases, or victims of violence, or people suddenly stricken). The staff on emergency services therefore is geared to give immediate emergency service to prevent death whenever possible. Many emergency services, especially in large cities, are also organized for frequent deaths, especially on weekends. At such times, the recovering (or non-sick) patients sometimes tend to receive scant attention, unless the service is flexibly organized for handling both types of patients. This patient competition also occurs on wards where patients die slowly. On the cancer ward, for example, when a patient nears death, sometimes he may unwittingly compete with other patients for nurses' or physicians' attention, several of whom may give care to the critically ill patient. When the emergency is over, or the patient dies, then the nurses may return to less immediately critical patients, reading their vital signs, managing treatments, and carrying out other important tasks. Mrs. Abel faired poorly in such competition with other patients during her long stay in the hospital, and especially during her last days.

All these temporal features of terminal care make for a complex organization of professional activity. The required organization is rendered even more complex by certain other matters involving temporality. Thus, what may be conveniently termed the "experiential careers" of patients, families, and staff members are very revelant to the action around dying patients. Some patients are very familiar with their diseases, but even than are encountering symptoms for the first time, such as Mrs. Abel confronting her intense pain. What a patient knows about the course of his disease, from previous experience with it, is very relevant to what will happen as he lies dying in the hospital. The same may be said about personnel in attendance upon him. Some personnel may be well acquainted with the predominant disease patterns found on their particular wards; but some may be newcomers to these diseases, although quite possible old hands with other illnesses. The newcomers may be quite unprepared for sudden changes of symptoms and vital signs, hence may be taken quite by surprise at crucial junctures: that is, they make bad errors in timing their actions. More experienced personnel are less likely to be cought unprepared, and are readier with appropriate care at each phase of the illness.

"Experiential careers" also refers to differential experiences that people have had with hospitals. Some patients return repeatedly to the same hospital ward, so that when the familiar face appears the staff may, for instance, be so shocked at the patient's deterioration, thinking "now he is going to die," that they react differently than they would to someone whom they do not know. Likewise, a patient who is unfamiliar with the ways of hospitals, or with this particular hospital, may react quite differently during the course of his dying than a patient who is familiar with the hospital. Mrs. Abel, though having repeated hospitalizations, was relatively new at the last hospital. She had been there once before. In short, both the hospital careers and illness careers of all parties to the dying situation may be of considerable importance, affecting both interaction around the dying patient, and the organization of his terminal care.

One type of experience is immensely relevant: we may conveniently refer to it as the differential "personal careers" of the interactants in the dying situation. This term simply underscores the more personal aspects of the iteraction. Thus, young nurses and physicians tend to react with immense involvement to the deaths of young terminal patients—much more so, generally, than toward elderly patients —for their identification with people of their own age was great.

Similarly, when an older woman reminds a young nurse of her own diseased mother, her actions toward the patient can be much affected. Mrs. Abel's young doctor was most touched by the similarity of her case to his mother's.

Among the most relevant reactions in the dying situation are personal conceptions of time. Thus, an elderly patient recognizing his approaching death may welcome it after a long and satisfying life, and may wish to review that life publicly; but his wife or nurse may refuse to listen, telling him that he should not give up hope of living or even cautioning him against being "so morbid." Other patients may throw the staff into turmoil because they will not accept their deaths: non-acceptance sometimes signifies that patients are protesting against destiny for cheating them of unfinished work—even when they are elderly. Such personalized conceptions of different persons in the dying situation may not only run counter to each other, they may also run counter to the staff's "work time," as for instance, when a patient's personal conception prevents the nurse from completing scheduled actions. Mrs. Abel's conceptions of time were continually at variance with the staff's.

One further class of events attending the course of dying is of crucial importance for the action around the dying patient. These events are the characteristic work of medical and hospital organization for the dying process. That the person is actually dying must be recognized in order that he be acted to as a dying person. At some point, others, and even he himself, may recognize that there now "is nothing more to do," nothing whatever. When he is nearing death, then a death watch usually takes place. When he dies, there must be a formal pronouncement and then an announcement to the family. At each point in time, actions are affected and—in terms of work— the staff's interrelated actions must be properly organized. In Mrs. Abel's case, much of this routine work was spared the cancer staff by her leaving the ward for an operation which ended in her death.

Taken all together, then, the total organization of activity—which we call "work"—during the course of dying is profoundly affected by temporal considerations. Some of these are obvious to almost everyone, some are not, and some are invisible, unless chance or voluntary admission brings them to others' attention. The entire web of temporal interrelationships we refer to as the *temporal order*. This includes the continual readjustment and coordination of staff effort which previously we termed the *temporal organization of work*. Our theoretical commentary weaves the complexity of this temporal order for Mrs. Abel's case.

9

Accountable and Non-Accountable Aspects of Terminal Care:
Much of organization of work in hospitals is guided by canons of
professional responsibility rather than by specific institutional and
legal rules. While it is true that many actions are governed by such
rules, considerable freedom is allowed nursing and medical personnel to accomplish their tasks. They are allowed this freedom first
of all, because they are trained professionals and presumed to know
what they are doing. For example, although a nurse must report
back by word or in writing what medical and nursing procedures
she has carried out, she need not necessarily report how those procedures were carried out, particularly, their social psychological aspects .Furthermore, rules and accountability to superiors cannot
possibly cover all contingencies of nursing and medical action—
many actions are not governed by explicit rules. Indeed in some
hospitals, both extensiveness of rules and laxity of rules is tolerated
in the belief that care of the patient calls for a minimum of hard-and-
fast rules and a maximum of innovation. Also, in many hospitals,
the multiplicity of medical purpose and theory, as well as personal
investment, are recognized. Too rigid a set of rules would only cause
turmoil and affect the hospital's over-all efficiency. Such considerations, then, mean that personnel—and especially professional personnel are allowed considerable latitude in acting responsibly
without requisite reporting back of their specific actions to superiors.
It is within these areas of latitude that Mrs. Abel's relationships with
staff disintegrated, went unnoticed and become nonaccountable actions for the staff.

Before we briefly explore the details of nonaccountability, it will
be useful to note aspects of medical and nursing action for which
personnel tend to be institutionally responsible. For example, the
terminal patients must be properly diagnosed and treated by the
physician and competently cared for by the nursing staff. In American hospitals, everything must be done to keep patients reasonably
free from physical pain. Physicians must make the decisions whether
or not to tell patients of their impeding death. Families must be
notified when death is near. Physicians must pronounce the patient
dead, and they, or a delegated person, must announce this fact to
the family. Nurses are responsible for post-mortem procedures until
the body is transferred from their jurisdiction. These actions are all
delegated, carried out, and reported upon. Personnel are accountable
institutionally and sometimes legally for geting these things done.

They are not nearly so accountable, however, for how they do
these things. In fact, little professional training is given for many
aspects of terminal care. As we noted before, medical students are
usually not taught how to announce death to relatives. They are not

10

taught how to tell the patient either, although as internes they quickly learn the dangers of telling certain patients. Nurses are taught how to give excellent physical care, but are not taught many of the details of working around dying patients. "Working around" in this instance includes the delicate psychological interplay which may occur between a terminal patient and the nurse. For Mrs. Abel this interplay was brutal. In general, the social and psychological (or "human") aspects of care are far less accountable than the more technical or procedural aspects.

While most nonaccountable (or little accountable) action consists of the acts of individuals, two or more personnel may also engage in such action, as in Mrs. Abel's case. For instance, two nursing aides may decide to handle a patient in a certain way but do not tell the head nurse. There is also what may be termed *ad hoc* accountability. With respect to many terminal patients, there evolves a great deal of institutionalized activity which includes both the what and the how, as well as both the medical and the psychological aspects of care. A patient, for instance, may become a vexing problem, and the entire staff may talk over ways of working with him. Into the staff's deliberations may enter much shrewdness and experience with similar patients. When this happens, what might otherwise have been a number of "invisible" actions now becomes more visibly a part of the ward's organized effort. When the patient dies or is transferred to another ward, this temporary organization and accountability of effort will disappear, as it did with Mrs. Abel.

There are two important points which we wish to underline about both accountable and less accountable action. The first is this: both kinds of activity are immensely relevant to the total interaction toward and around the dying patient. By this, we mean not merely that the less institutionalized, less visible behavior must be noted by any researcher, but also that much of what most physicians and nurses would term "good terminal care" falls on the nonaccountable side of the ledger.

The second point is that both accountable and less or non-accountable action are linked intimately with the temporal organization of work. It scarcely seems necessary to elaborate this point here: one need only think of the differential behavior called forth as a patient comes closer to death. Then a typical non-accountable situation is that the relatives ask the nurse a series of questions, and she answers them in a fashion that seems sensible to her. She is not likely to report her conversation to the head nurse, except possibly to note their general state of mind by a characterizing phrase or two ("they were terribly anxious.") This temporality of action—whether more or less

11

accountable—is of the utmost significance in understanding what happens during the entire course of the patient's dying. For example, the temporal organization of care for Mrs. Abel continually enforced more and more isolation upon her as she neared death. The staff were nonaccountable for such a situation and its consequences.

DYING TRAJECTORIES

The dying trajectory of each patient has at least two outstanding properties. First, it takes place over time: it has *duration*. There can be much variation in duration among specific trajectories, ranging from instant death to months, as for Mrs. Abel. Second, a trajectory has *shape:* it can be graphed. It plunges straight down; it moves slowly downward (Mrs. Abel); it vacilates slowly, moving slightly up and down before diving radically downward; it moves slowly down at first, then hits a long plateau, then plunges abruptly to death.

Neither duration nor shape is a purely objective psychological property. They are perceived properties; their dimensions depend on *when* the perceiver initially *defines* someone as dying and on his expectations of how that dying will proceed. Dying trajectories are, then, (as noted earlier) *perceived courses of dying,* rather than the actual courses themselves. This distinction is readily evident in the type of trajectory which involves a short reprieve from death. This reprieve represents an unexpected deferment of death. On the other hand, a lingering death may mean that bystanders expect faster dying, as in Mrs. Abel's trajectory.

Since dying patients enter hospitals at varying distances from death, and are defined in terms of when and how they will die, various types of trajectories are commonly recognized by the hospital personnel. For instance, there is the trajectory that is a complete surprise: a patient who is expected to recover suddenly dies. A frequently found trajectory on emergency wards is the expected swift death. Many patients are brought in because of fatal accidents, and nothing can be done to prevent their deaths. Expected lingering while dying is another type of trajectory; it is characteristic, for example, of cancer patients like Mrs. Abel. Besides the short-term reprieve, there may also be the suspended-sentence trajectory. Another commonly recognized pattern is entry-reentry: the patient, slowly going downhill, returns home several times between stays at the hospital. All these generalized types of trajectories rest upon the perceivers' expectations of "duration" and "shape."

Regardless of the particular attributes of a specific patient's trajectory, there are ordinarily certain events—we shall term them

12

"critical junctures"—which appear along the dying trajectory and are directly handled by the temporal organization of hospital work. These occur either in full or truncated form: (1) The patient is defined as dying; (2) Staff and family then make preparations for his death, as he may himself if he knows he is dying; (3) At some point, there seems to be "nothing more to do" to prevent death; (4) The final descent may take weeks, or days, or merely hours, ending in (5) the "last hours," (6) the death watch, and (7) death itself. Somewhere along his course of dying, there may be announcements that the patient is dying, or that he is entering or leaving a phase of dying. After death, death itself must be legally pronounced, and then publicly announced.

When these critical junctures occur as expected, on schedule, then all participants—including the patient, sometimes—are prepared for their occurance—the work involved is provided for and integrated by the temporal order of the hospital. For instance, the nurses are ready for a death watch when they can anticipate approximately when the patient will be very near death. When, however, critical junctures are not expected or are off schedule, staff members and family alike are caught off guard, or at least somewhat unprepared. This case will offer many examples both of anticipated and unanticipated junctures. The point we wish to emphasize here is that expectations are crucial to the way critical junctures are handled by all involved. For that reason we turn next to a discussion of death expectations.

EXPECTATIONS OF DEATH

When a person enters a hospital, one of the most important initial questions is, "What's the diagnosis?" This question is no less important when the patient is fated soon to die, unless death is so imminent that diagnosis is pointless. What is done to and for most patients depends mainly on the answer to the diagnostic and its allied prognostic questions. Modern hospitals are organized to insure relatively speedy answers. If initial diagnosis is uncertain, additional soundings are typically made, and the course of the illness itself, during the next few days, may prompt more accurate answers.

As we remarked earlier, many a hospital patient (and Mrs. Abel is one) poses for the staff two questions simultaneously: Is this patient going to die here, and, if so, when? The first of these questions refers to "uncertainty of death" while the second refers to "time of death." Even more specifically, let us say that relative certainty of death means the degree to which the defining person (physician,

13

nurse, or even the patient himself) is convinced that the patient will die. Let us say that time of death means the expectation of either (a) when the certain death will occur, or (b) when the uncertainty about death will be resolved. Time units can range from minutes to months, varying with the nature of the illness and the patient's location in the hospital. For example, on emergency wards only a few minutes may pass before it is known for certain whether patient will live. About premature babies, nurses usually think of death in terms of hours or a few days at most. For cancer patients the time unit may be months.

In combination, certainty and time yield four types of "death expectations": (1) certain death at a known time, (2) certain death at an unknown time, (3) uncertain death but a known time when the question will be resolved, and (4) uncertain death and unkown time when the question will be resolved. As we shall show, in the following chapters, these expectations have varying effects on the interaction of nurses and physicians with Mrs. Abel.

Anyone may read the medical signs and draw his own conclusions, the terminal patient included. But in American hospitals, the attending physician is the only one who can legitimately define the patient's condition, because of his professional expertise and the professional mandate that he be medically responsible for the patient. Ordinarily, only he may tell patients they are dying. Under extraordinary conditions, nurses tell patients or relatives directly, but this is not the usual practice, and definitely not the practice in Mrs. Abel's case.

But nurses, too, must correctly assess whether the patient is dying and when he will die. To make those assessments is often no easy matter. The nurses were behind the physician in assessing Mrs. Abel's dying condition. In forming their expectations, the nurses may rely on their own reading of cues—how the patient looks and acts, what his charts report about him—as well as on cues flashed, perhaps unwittingly or obliquely, by the doctor. Sometimes they also receive direct information from the doctor; typically, they trust this source more than their own individual or collective reading of cues, although the reverse may be true if they are experienced nurses and the doctor seems inexperienced, incompetent, or not well acquainted with the case. Sometimes the cues are so obvious that the physician needs to say little or nothing. So, although the most legitimate source for forming and expressing death expectations is the physician, the nurses also observe cues constantly.

Doctors vary considerably as to whether they give nurses a legitimate basis for death expectations. ("The doctor may or may not tell us a patient is critical. We decide. They expect us to use our beans.")

14

It is unusual for a nurse to ask the doctor directly, but there may be an implicit understanding that he will tell her, or she can hint that he should tell her or give her cues. He may tell her obliquely at first, but more directly when the patient nears death. In one Catholic hospital a nurse told us: "There is no formal declaration that a patient is terminal. Sometimes a doctor will tell the nurse, but usually you just pick it up." She added: "If the doctor knows that a patient is going to die, I prefer to know it." This nurse wants legitimate expectations, but she is forced to rely mainly on cues, as with Mrs. Abel. Sometimes nothing much needs to be said, as when a cancer patient who has returned often to the service returns now in obviously critical condition, and everyone, residents and nurses alike, agree that "this is the last time." Sometimes the cues are as explicit as words might be, as when a feeble patient who might to the inexperienced still seem to have a chance to live is taken off intravenous blood injections.

Two principal types of cues that the nurses can read are the patient's physical condition and the temporal references made either by themselves or the medical staff. Physical cues, ranging from those that spell hope to those that indicate immediate death, generally establish the certainty aspect of death expectations. Temporal cues, however, have many reference points. A major one is the typical progression of the disease, against which the patient's actual movement is measured (he is "going fast" or "lingering"). Another is the doctor's expectation about how long the patient will remain in the hospital. For instance, one patient's hospitalization was "lasting longer" than the short stay anticipated by the physician. Work schedules also provide a temporal reference: nurses adjust their expectations according to whether the patient can continue being bathed, turned, fed, and given sedation regularly. All such references pertain to the temporal aspect of dying—to how long the patient is expected to live.

Because physical cues are generally easier to read and their presence helps to establish some degree of certainty about dying, temporal cues are rather indeterminate when the physical ones are absent. The patient may die "sometime" or "at any time." As both types of cues accumulate, they may support each other; for example, as Mrs. Abel's physical condition became more grave her hospitalization grew longer. But physical and temporal cues can also cancel each other: thus, an unduly long hospitalization can be balanced or even negated by increasingly hopeful physical cues. When cues cancel each other, nurses can use the more hopeful one (he is going home sooner than expected) to balance or deny the less hopeful (he looks bad). As physical and temporal cues accumulate faster and become more severe, they become harder to deny, and the expectation of death is gradually more firmly established.

Nurses' definitions of the patient's illness status—that is, their expectations—affect their behavior toward him. Therefore, the particular moment when their expectations change is significant. For example, even when the physician's cues imply that the patient is doomed, as when he stops blood transfusions, the nurses may still not be absolutely sure that the implied prediction is accurate. They may not lower their levels of alertness or reduce their efforts to save the patient. They may say of the patient, as one nurse did, "If he comes out of it, we'll work on him. He only has to give us the slightest cue." Since the doctor has said nothing official, even nurses who believe the patient is dying can still give him an outside chance and standy ready to save him. They remain constantly alert to counter-cues. "Everybody is simply waiting," said one nurse. If the doctor had indicated that the patient would die within the day, nurses would have ceased their constant watch for countercues and reduced their efforts to save him, concentrating instead on giving comfort to the last, with no undue prolonging of life. When the nurses realized that Mrs. Abel would die on their ward their behavior changed to isolating her.

Indeed the changing expectations of nurses and physicians actually map out the patient's changes of status. Many patterns of "status passage," with typical rates of movement, are well known. A classical pattern is the lingering patient: he is certain to die, but when he will do so is unknown, and he does not die for some while. On one cancer ward we studied, an all too-typical sequence of expectations for the lingering patient ran the gamut of various stages of determinancy: from original prognosis of certain death but uncertain time, through the weeks when the patient began obviously to decline, to the time when his precise time of death finally became relatively certain. Before the final decline takes place, such patients may alternate between hospital visits and periods at home. Often the nurses feel that a lingering patient is taking more time than is proper, because there is really no hope for him. (In this sense, even an unknown time period has limits.)

A patient expected to die on schedule, but who suddenly begins to recover slightly or to linger—the short-term reprieve pattern— can cause problems for nurses, family, physicians, and hospital administrators. Here is an example: One patient who was expected to die within four hours had no money, and needed a special machine in order to last longer. A private hospital, at which he had been a frequent paying patient for thirty years, agreed to receive him as a charity patient. He did not die immediately but started to linger

16

indefinitely, even to the point where there was some hope that he might live. The money problem, however, created much concern among both his family members and the hopsital administrators. Paradoxically, the doctor had continually to reassure both parties that this patient, who actually lasted six weeks, would soon die; that is, to try to change their expectations back to "certain to die on time."

Another pattern, which may be called the vacillating pattern, is a variation on the short-term reprieve. The patient alternates from "certain to die on time" to "lingering." The alternating may occur sufficiently often to cause stress among family members and hos pital personnel. Whenever the patient genuinely starts to fade, the nurses may call the family, for, as one nurse said, "If you do not call the family and the patients die, that's wrong." The family members arrive for their last look at the dying man, but he begins to linger. They finally leave saying, "please call us again" when he begins to die. Family and nurses may go repeatedly through this stressful cycle. The physician and the chaplain may also be affected. Changes in the activities and moods of the various participants are thus linked with this vacillating pattern, and the nurses' mood is typically one of relief when at last they can forecast the end of the unusual lingering, or as with Mrs. Abel, a departure from the ward.

The two extremes toward which patients move are "getting well" or "certain to die at a specific time," but nurses and physicians may have other, intermediate expectations for a given patient who leaves the hospital. He may have arrived with uncertain prognosis, but is being sent home diagnosed as cancerous: certain to die, but "when" is quite unknown. The prognosis of more puzzling cases may be uncertain on both counts.

The staff may be surprised by unexpected changes in the expected passage of patients toward death. Among the most surprising changes are the sudden death, or onset of death, of a patient who previously had prognosis of doubtful certainty and time. Of course, the surprise is greatest when there has been no death expectation whatever, as when seemingly healthy or recovering patients die. When such patients die on the operating table, the impact is tremendous. The patient's death is too sudden: there is no time to prepare for it. In one instance, a surgeon much admired by his nursing staff shocked them with an unexpected loss on the operating table. Rumors of negligence were rife, until autopsy showed that the man had died of unanticipated natural causes. In less traumatic instances, when expectations are revised as the patient moves toward death, but his progress turns out to be unusual, personnel may experience a disquieting feeling of having missed certain steps. Few nurses, however, were disquieted about missing Mrs. Abel's death.

When the staff closely approximates a dying patient's trajectory, its work with other patients, as well as with him, is made easier. Critical junctures during his dying can be planned for so that manpower, for instance, will not be withdrawn suddenly from other patients nor the scheduling of tasks with them be disrupted. Miscalculations in forecasting or perceiving trajectories can play havoc with the organization of work—as when one or more patients unexpectedly and swiftly begin to die. Each service usually has routine procedures for managing occasional expectable emergencies, but this organizational machinery may not be sufficient to cope with crisis stemming from gross miscalculations of trajectory. As we shall see, when such crises occur, the staff attempts, as quickly as possible, to regain control over the organization of work. Since a revised notion of the patient's condition may necessitate new procedures or additional time spent at his bedside, considerable re-ordering of work—even changes of the division of labor—may be involved.

Disruption of the ward's organization of work is paralleled by a shattering of its characteristic "sentimental order"—that intangible but very real patterning of mood and sentiment which characteristically exists on each ward. For instance, in an intensive care unit where cardiac patients die frequently the sentimental order is relatively unaffected by one more speedy death; but if a hopeless patient such as Mrs. Abel lingers on and on the sentimental as well as work order is profoundly affected. A much different instance may help to convey the same point: On obstetrics servivces, the characteristic sentimental order is one of relative cheer and optimism. When a delivering mother unexpectedly dies, the characteristic chaos which follows is a visible sign of the shattered normal sentimental pattern.

In sum, the lingering trajectory exemplified by Mrs. Abel's case is an important, poignant case history which illustrates in detail one of the many typical kinds of dying trajectories covered by our theory. Now let us procede to see the lingering, dying trajectory in detail.

Chapter II

THE DEATH

Mrs. Abel is the central character in this case history of a lingering trajectory. She was a middle-aged married woman, with a rather ineffectual husband who plays only a minor role in the story of her trajectory. She entered the cancer service of the hospital in November, briefly stayed a while, and then returned never to leave until she died in February. As will be seen, she suffered from a great deal of pain, which increased as she declined. At first she seems to everyone, including the researchers, merely to be a patient who was in some or much pain. Later everyone understands that this patient probably will die and quite possibly during her current stay at this hospital.

Even before the patient began to decline, the nursing staff had found her a most difficult charge, and tended to spend as little time with her as possible. Weeks before she finally died, she experienced virtual isolation. The staff members could neither suffer her nor withstand the ordeal through which she was going and in which they were participating. Her death finally occurred after even the most empathetic nurse had pulled away and her physician had, because of his own helplessness, abandoned her to a last-ditch but improbable and quite possibly fatal surgical operation. Mrs. Abel understood the riskiness of this operation but was almost beyond caring. She could neither stand her almost unendurable pain nor derive much bitterness from the almost total isolation which staff had imposed on her. Surgery represented to her more of a potential release from her impossible situation than a chance to live—if live it really was, since she foresaw herself as "a vegetable"—a bit longer.

The story of the trajectory actually will be told somewhat in reverse. It begins with its ending, as Mrs. Abel's death and the immediately preceding events are described. In the initial account, we shall see that important tertiary themes (along with the four substories) already appear. One is the relative autonomy of hospital

19

services and the resultant minimal communication among the services —poignantly illustrated by the circumstances under which the operation was carried out, and the relative ignorance of the patient by the surgeons, as well as that of the cancer ward staff about what the surgeons thought the operation was all about. Another subsidiary theme is the fateful progressive deterioration of relationships between Mrs. Abel's physician and the ward personnel; this deterioration paralleled the downward course of Mrs. Abel's own relationships. A third theme is about how medical technology is now able to keep patients alive far beyond where life perhaps makes much sense. The relief of the staff after Mrs. Abel's death is related to the tension which often builds up around lingering deaths prolonged by efficient technological means—prolonged unnecessarily as seen by the staff itself. This is an issue which is beginning to become not merely a professional but a public issue. A fourth theme is the inadequacy of current nursing and medical practice, as taught even in the most advanced professional schools, for handling cases like Mrs. Abel. Perhaps the chaplain's eventual pulling away in helplessness from Mrs. Abel indicates most clearly the failure of professional education to prepare practitioners for coping successfully with such patients. A fifth theme is that dying occurs within an organizational context: Mrs. Abel is only one of a number of patients whom the staff must simultaneously care for and work with. What happens to her cannot be understood without understanding the hospital as an organization for work.

STORY: THE DEATH

SY: I saw Mrs. Abel last Monday (the 17th of February), and she was looking forward to surgery: "I hope I die." I realized she saw it as a "way out," not only in terms of pain but also as a way of dying. It might be difficult to separate the two but this was before she saw the lobotomy operation as stopping pain.

Unfortunately I did not get to see her before surgery although I told her that I was going to be with her the following day—that is, the day of surgery. So I went up later at 7:30 and she had already been moved. I went to the operating room and tried to let her know I was there, but don't think she caught it.

The operating room nurse who had come to take Mrs. Abel to the operating room was very angry with the nursing staff because the patient was on a low bed, and the orderly and she had struggled very hard to get the patient onto the operating room guerney. Mrs. Abel had not been changed. Ordinarily, these kinds of things would be taken care of for any patient going to surgery. The operating room nurse was very angry because the nursing staff there was busy passing out trays and other things, knowing the operating room people were busy struggling to get this patient onto the guerney. Finally, in anger, the operating room nurse hollered for help. Although the patient was very drowsy, the operating room staff said she was crying about the pain because of the movement involved. When they got her to the operating room, the nurses said about fifteen or twenty minutes were involved in moving this patient to her position on the operating room table. I asked what they thought about Mrs. Abel. "Good God, I pity the nurse who has to take care of this patient." I said I had been taking care of this patient, and they said, "No kidding," in other words they thought how horrible—because any nurse would have a terrible time taking care of her.

When I heard this I thought, "How sad for this patient. If she dies on the table, or if she dies without regaining consciousness, this is her last interaction with people—which is typical of her interaction throughout her life . . ." Before Mrs. Abel went under anesthesia she said, *"I hope I die."* I realized, or it reinforced my feeling, that she saw the surgery not only as a way to stop pain, but as a means of dying. This is what the nurse there said to me. I asked, 'What did she say before she went?" Those were the last words Mrs. Abel said before she went under.

Then, shortly after, the physician or the surgeon came in to scrub the patient's head and do a further shave and I thought, "My God, the only thing she ever had any pride in was her hair, and this is being stripped." This was Mrs. Abel's crowning point . . .

During the surgery there was a lot of interchange between resident and intern about what was going on, the procedures involved; the intern was being taught how to do these things. I thought, "Well, she's dying, the research patient."

At 11:30 they ran into trouble. Up to this time there was no change in vital signs and she was pretty good. I couldn't believe it because I thought that something would happen at an earlier stage. Actually, though, they ran into trouble because of the actual manipulation of the brain rather than the vital signs. At this point they called in the chief, and it was then that I left.

At 3:30 I went back to the operating room and the patient was still there. They said it might take about an hour or so. So at 4:30 I went back, and the patient was in the recovery room. She was not responding at all. I called her several times but she did not answer. The recovery room nurse said her vital signs were very poor. Blood pressure was running 80 over 30. One pupil was fixed and not re-acting. Her color was terrible, her whole body was edematous. I realized the patient wasn't going to make it. She probably wasn't going to be conscious again. The recovery room nurse thought the patient wasn't going to make it and felt perhaps it would be a good thing. Then she said, "You know, I looked at the patient's breast and saw her arm, and I almost fell over because it was so awful." Later, I checked again, and the patient wasn't making any progress. Her vital signs were bad. I realized that she *really* wasn't going to make it.

I went to the ICU to make arrangements to take care of the pa-tient. The head nurse said, "No." I didn't want to argue: I thought, "If Mrs. Abel does make it, which I doubt, she will be so miserable to care for that they will *welcome* my going in to take care of her."

AS: Did the head nurse on the ICU know who the patient was?

SY: No. The other thing was that I assumed the patient would go to ICU; but when I went down there and asked about Mrs. Abel coming down, they said she was not scheduled to come to the ICU. This is when I felt the neurologist had a very different estimate of the patient's physical state.

AS: Why did she go in for the operation—what kind of opera-tion was it?

SY: Surgery to control pain. It's called hypophysectomy.

SA: The surgeon denied this operation is done for pain, so I pushed him about it. I talked with Dr. Foote, the intern who ac-tually shaved her head the first night, though he was not in on sur-gery that morning. He agreed with her physician that this surgery is done for reduction of the growth of tumor which secondarily re-duces pain, particularly if there have been bone metastases. I push-ed him with a description of a similar case when I took care of a woman who immediately perked up. I had watched the dramatic pain relief of this woman (from narcotics every four hours around the clock, to my giving her a sixth amount of dosage only once dur-ing the first four-hour period immediately post-operative). She was carried on aspirin from then on until she died. This procedure was done specifically for pain and for no other reason. I was pushing him, and he was still denying this was done for pain, but rather for reduction of her tumor growth. She was such a bad risk—for when I talked to her physician, Dr. Colp, today he said that when he first asked them two to three weeks ago she was in fair condition. But the day of surgery she was half dead before she went to surgery. He said, "I guess they are used to working on half dead patients in

22

terms of neurosurgery, so they didn't care. Their average statistics, "mortality rates," are pretty poor anyway.

AS: Why did they bother with the operation when they knew she would die within a week or two at most?

SY: I got a different impression in talking to Dr. Pitt, the intern on the case. He said the patient's vital signs and the other studies prior to surgery weren't good, but she seemed like a pretty good risk.

SA: They didn't do any electrolyte studies.

SY: They *didn't*.

SA: They *didn't*. Because Dr. Colp did not order them, and they weren't done. He said he thought she was in good potassium balance because he had been feeding her potassium like crazy and so purposely didn't add to it. He didn't think there was any value in doing so. He said, "I don't think *anybody* is going to raise an eyebrow or criticize the hospital. The husband is happy, we're happy, everybody it happy."

AS: Who made the actual decision to send her to operation?

SY and SA: (together) The neurosurgeons.

SA: Didn't you say that Dr. Colp had actually questioned this decision at the last minute?

SY: Yes, he wanted to be sure that the patient knew the risks in terms of not having a 100% cure or relief of pain. He said this to her, over and over and over again: "Did the neurologist say this to you?"

SA: The surgeons denied this operation was being done for pain, except that this is the reason they gave to the patient. This is the reason the head nurse gave this afternoon when I asked, "Why was the surgery done?" She said, "For relief of pain." This is what they had been told, too.

AS: So this is what you believed, too, Shizu?

SY: At first I didn't believe it because this is not what I had been told. It didn't make sense to me, because in the first recording I made, I felt very strongly about this. It was after talking with Dr. Pitt that I felt maybe this was true.

AS: I'm still confused about *why* the neurosurgeons made the decision to operate.

SA: I haven't been able to get to Dr. Wallace yet. He's the neurosurgeon who made the decision.

AS: Then we'd better find out on what basis the decision was made.

SA: The intern, Dr. Foote, described her as a bad case, and I asked, 'What do you mean by a bad case?" He said her metastasis was incurable. There was no hope of doing anything about it anyway.

Then he described Mrs. Abel's ambivalence about death: "I shaved her head last night; one minute she was asking to die on the table, and in the next breath she's asking me how long it would take for her hair to grow in. This is the same kind of ambivalence that you see with many people near death."

AS: Did he indicate anything by his manner, in talking with you, how he felt?

SA: That she would not live long enough for it to make any difference whether her hair grew out or not. What he did say was that she will wear a skull cap, or something or other, to make her look pretty during that time. But he didn't expect her to live.

SY: When I was in the operating room I looked at her and thought, "She's dead." Her whole face looked as though she were dead—the color—it was like a death mask. You know how when the head is shaven—just the face—that's the way she looked. I really felt terrible for her because she had made no positive relationship with anybody, and she must have felt that everybody abandoned her—her husband, everybody. Because I felt so badly about it, when she was in the recovery room I made it a point to say to the nurse up there that should Mrs. Abel become conscious, please tell her that I was in surgery and had been by to see her, so that this last contact was going to be made. But the patient did not regain consciousness.

At 10:30 the patient was sent to ICU; the recovery room closes at 11:00. Two hours later I had been told the patient died. The following morning when I went up to the recovery room, they said she had passed away. So I caught Dr. Pitt, the one who had scrubbed in on surgery—the man who said he felt the patient did not seem such a bad risk. I asked if the patient had regained consciousness enough to say anything about pain. "No, she was too far gone to respond in any way." I asked if the hypophysectomy was done for pain and he said, "Yes." This is *his* impression. Then he immediately went into a discussion of did I want "to go down to see the autopsy" which was being done? He said that the cause of death, although cardiac arrest, was probably from multiple causes because she was extremely edematous, and he began to list all these causes. I bowed out of the autopsy because I didn't think I could tolerate it.

Then I went up to the cancer unit. They had already heard about the patient's death. There were statements like, "Isn't it sad," "Isn't it terrible," *but* "It was the best thing in the long run." They were interested in the pathology when I said an autopsy was being done. They dwelt mostly on wanting to find out what the pathology was: "Be sure and come back and let us know what they found."

AS: What would you say was their general mood?

SY: A general mood of relief. I felt relief, too. I didn't think there was any sadness. The discussion with Dr. Pitt was dispassionate.

AS: Did you pick up spontaneous remarks from the nurses— off the top of their heads?

SY: No, just "isn't it sad," "it's terrible." Did you get that impression, Shirley?

SA: They aren't talking about it at all. They are very quiet, and what little discussion there is, is in terms of the disease entity itself. However, there is a difference in their relationship—this is the first day I've seen the head nurse smile. And they're talking to me again, finally. It's the first she's spent any time with me at all. This is true of Mrs. Hand declining before to tell me anything about the operating procedure or why it was done. She said, "I know, but I think I'd better let one of the other nurses tell you." There's a real sense of . . . like somebody had taken a millstone or weight from everyone's neck—from the chaplain, to the surgeons, to the physician—everybody involved. I think it was Dr. Foote who told me that probably there had not been any heroics. Dr. Colp told me they tried closed cardiac massage for fifteen minutes. He also gave me the information on the autopsy today. He stayed for almost everything. Death was actually from multiple causes. They've signed her out as a cardiac arrest, although it was only after that she stopped breathing.

SY: I talked to Dr. Colp over the phone and he assumed immediately that I was interested in the pathology of the patient. He described what you just described, then he expressed great relief and said that it was better for the husband and all the people involved, whom he listed, including himself.

SA: But he also said, "It's better for the nurses. There's more relief for the nurses than there is for me." He emphasized this the last couple of times I've seen him: that they had to put up with more.

AS: I take it there is a change of behavior toward you, Shirley, because now they are talking to you whereas before they progressively avoided you because they thought your speaking with Mrs. Abel made her more complaining. What about you, Shizu?

SY: They were happy when I first began taking care of Mrs. Abel. I was "in like Flynn," and they talked to me about Mrs. Abel. Then as her stay extended and her condition worsened, they avoided me more and more, and I had to seek them out more and more.

AS: What about now?

SY: Now I can't tell because there was just this one interaction, but they were anxious for me to come back and report. I said I would be back next week and they said "fine," so I guess this is an indication that they are now ready to talk to me.

One other thing about Dr. Colp: the last thing he said was he was not going to admit any more patients like this. They were all going to go to "City" and "County" (hospitals).

SA: He would never admit any one unless the patient actually requests the favor of his last few days of terminal care in this hospital. He frankly stated that with Mrs. Abel as a problem, and one other small incident, he had "had" it.

SY: One other thing: the social worker stated that they had tremendous difficulty when working with Dr. Colp in making discharge plans. He had great difficulty in releasing patients to the outside.

AS: Coming back to *your* remark, Shirley; "he had *had* it," you say. Meaning what?

SA: The problems involved in communicating with the staff.

AS: You mean he will have no more patients?

SA: He will admit no more patients to this hospital. He has his research projects, and he's staying another year to work on this research project. He has his clinic patients but will not admit any hospital patients.

I went to see Dr. Tree, the research physician, today. He wasn't there, but his secretary gave me the information I wanted: he didn't work with Mrs. Abel since Christmas because he was told the budget would not permit keeping this patient any longer. I said, "You mean, you didn't know the patient was still here?" And the secretary said, "No." I asked, "Did you know she died the other night?" She said, "No." I said, "She went to surgery on Tuesday and died Tuesday night." She said, "Well, that's probably for the best." This is the reason Dr. Tree was no longer in the picture.

SY: That's interesting. Did you say *after* Christmas? But the patient kept waiting for the arrival of Dr. Tree to continue his research.

AS: So he never said goodbye; he never terminated his visits?

SA: No, and he never terminated as far as the staff knew. All of a sudden the surgeon came into the picture, so that kept her in the hospital. Dr. Colp has told me in the last two weeks that since Christmas he had been planning to send her home and had worked out the details with the social worker, as far as even getting a nursing home, until the advent of the surgical procedure. And then she was maintained here.

SY: This is a very different story from the social worker's. She said, "All the plans were ready for the patient to go home, but Dr. Colp made it impossible for me to discharge the patient."

SA: Further, in relation to the floor's response I talked to day and evening shifts and got similar responses from both sets of nurses. When I made the comment, "It sort of seems strange up here without Mr. Abel on the floor," two of the nurses kind of laughed and one said, "Yeah, the last thing she did as they were taking her down the elevator was to be screaming about 'where's my pillow' "! That's the last that the staff saw of this patient. And so it seems like a strange atmosphere for them now.

AS: Have you any idea what they were doing while the patient was upstairs?

SA: They were sort of curious but relieved because this automatically meant she was off their floor. Automatically because Kai could hardly wait, the week before, when the operation was cancelled. She said, "We can hardly wait because she needs a new place to go, for her own sake"—meaning Mrs. Abel.

AS: They were already saying, weren't they, that, "We could no longer do any good for her"?

SA: They said this long ago, before Christmas, but Kai said it again when the renewed hope of actually getting rid of her came up —through surgery—getting her to another floor with another staff.

SY: Dr. Colp actually made this statement too.

AS: Was there any administrative reason why she could not have been moved to another floor *after* Dr. Tree gave up his research?

SA: She was never transferred because she remained under Dr Colp's service right to the end.

SY: I asked about the possibility of moving the patient if she got into a terminal state, and the head nurse said she didn't know about that but didn't think it was very fair—fair to the other staff who would get this patient.

SA: That was the supervisor's general feeling when I talked with her—not fair to another staff, and they should just leave things as they were until they could get rid of the patient from the hospital completely. It isn't fair to the patient either. But she said, "My staff comes first."

AS: What about the social worker?

SY: The social worker again expressed relief. She also had heard about the patient's death. I asked her how she thought the staff viewed herself, and she said the staff on the cancer unit knew the social worker as a person who got patients off the unit. "I was looked upon as the one to push her out." As it became evident Mrs. Abel was going to stay, the nurses began to view the social worker as another victim of circumstances and would make such statements as, "Well, you know how she is," indicating that one can't do much about it.

The social worker felt the patient actually wanted the surgery, and that the patient was getting very anxious from the delay because the operation was delayed three times: first for surgical repairs of the instruments; second because of the changed plans from lobotomy to hypophesectomy; and then the problem that was involved in getting blood for this patient, because she had had so many drugs that might enter into the action.

SA: When I saw the chaplain today, I said, "I've been trying to catch up with you. Where have you been?" He answered, "I was here all day yesterday," and started talking to me. "The day before, I took the day off. I decided I needed the day off." I said, "Oh." He went on, knowing that I wanted to talk about Mrs. Abel. I asked, "When did you see her?" He said, "Actually Friday was the last time I saw her prior to Tuesday." He had assigned her to one of his students, a man with maturity, whom he felt would grow from the experience of working with Mrs. Abel. This man was a Baptist. Mrs. Abel was not a Baptist.

Then he told me he wasn't sure whether she had made a confession to him as a person or not, but she had sort of changed her wayward religious ideas. (She had some very unorthodox beliefs about reincarnation which were bothering some nurses way back in the beginning. I had a philosophical discussion with her about this. So did *he* later on.) He thought that by the end she had come to some agreement with his more orthodox position about the meaning of life. He had a very good session with her on Friday.

He said, "When I went in, she obviously was very uncomfortable." Her position on the chair indicated a great deal of pain, and she said, "I'm looking for the nurses." He said to me, "I'd been pushing this just as hard as I could, and I was wondering how far I could go . . . I'd been an orderly before I went into the ministry in the hospital and worked in the operating room, and so forth . . . I thought I could do something for her." (And I asked, "You mean, we actually pushed you into nursing care?" He answered, "Yes. I've been in this business for 25 years.") So he said, "Is there something I could do for you, Mrs. Abel?" She agreed to have him straighten the pillows out and get her situated so she would be more comfortable. Her gown was awry and by the end, she hadn't really cared if he were in the room or not.

But she had asked him to pray, and pray that she would die on the table. "I thought about it for a minute and realized here is a woman who is undergoing a lot of suffering, who cannot tolerate suffering. Her suffering tolerance is pretty low, and so I prayed that if this was within the will of God, that she might die." She had said, "I know I'm dying." (I told him, "Yes, she had known this for about a week and a half, that she was in a terminal stage.") So he went on, "I prayed that if she was going to go anyway, that if this might be the will of God, that she die on the table." She was very quiet and accepted this when he was praying. He said this was actually the best session the two of them had ever had. There was "real communication" and feeling between them. "I went away feeling rather good about it." When he started to leave he asked her, "Is there something else you would like the nurses to do for you?" She said, "Yes, see that one comes immediately." He said to me, "I wasn't sure I could but said 'yes' anyway." So he caught up with Kai in the hallway, put his arm around her and said, "How about doing me a favor. Would you go in and take care of Mrs. Abel immediately?" Kai replied, "I was just finishing one patient and going on to another. Yes, I'll do it for you as a favor."

I asked the chaplain if he had run into this "intolerance" business with the nurses, "a little." He was just beginning to feel this in their behavior to himself. That's why he didn't know whether they would do it for him or not. But he was using this tactic as a kind of leverage.

I asked him, "Well, how do you feel? Do you feel relief?"

"Yes, there was nothing we could do for her. It's probably best that she died. Everybody was so frustrated and having so many problems, even me." He had a lot of feelings, *before,* about nurses being unable to cope with this situation and not having insight into what was going on. And he said, "You know, this woman, who all of us thought was so transparent, was really opaque. We really didn't know her."

SY: My discussion with the chaplain was the same as yours. He said he was quite frustrated with the problem. Then he immediately began to relate similar kinds of experiences where he had met with success.

AS: He's the only person who got any kind of closure at all, that I can see; and his was only partial. But he did get some closure on Friday and some minimum satisfaction with Mrs. Abel by partially converting the woman away from her "wayward religious ideas."

SY: He didn't express the same degree of satisfaction when I talked to him because I talked to him earlier. He said that he never felt that he got through to her.

AS: You should check out why he didn't see her after Friday.

SA: He said, "I sent a student in."

AS: Why didn't *he* go?

SY: I found out the theology student who saw her, and I'm going to catch him on Monday.

AS: Any information on the husband?

SY: No, I couldn't get any information. I asked the recovery room nurses, and they said, "No, no one seems to have seen the husband."

SA: The husband was in the night before surgery, because when the doctor went into her room to shave her head the husband was there. He said the husband didn't really talk to him about this, and about the fact that she was losing her hair. The husband made no response to the hair.

AS: But he showed up, at last.

SA: Yes, he showed up again. Well, I had seen him once. Shizu had seen him once with the social worker. So that's three times we know of.

THEORETICAL COMMENTARY: THE DEATH

Mrs. Abel's death simultaneously ended both a lengthy, arduous dying trajectory and a hospital career. Her surgery merely constituted the last stage of a hospital career. This career had provided a dying trajectory which in the end left few viable alternatives. Surgery was a "way out" of an intolerable ordeal for Mrs. Abel, her doctor, and the nursing staff of the cancer ward. For some time there had been nothing-more-to-do for her; and her doctor, urged on by the nursing staff and social worker, had reached the point of doing or trying anything that might relieve the patient of her pain, her discomfort, and mitigate her isolation; that would relieve the nursing staff of a patient they could no longer tolerate; and that would relieve the hospital of a non-paying patient. She had reached a point of pain, physical degeneration and social isolation which indicated that her current hospital career—being provided comfort until death or discharge—no longer was tenable. Yet the patient lived on, alert to her dying and pain, crying for relief and attention.

Accordingly, her doctor decided to alter the end of her career. Neuro-surgery was prescribed for a variety of reasons and purposes, none of which were clearly affirmed. The purposes comprised, as far as we could grasp later, pain relief, tumor reduction, providing a mode of death for the patient, research, training and practice for the neurosurgeons and getting the patient off the ward for the relief of the nursing staff and her doctor. The possibility of death was acknowledged by all, including the patient. The degree of risk was variously appraised and admitted. The outcome was death within hours after surgery. The death was met with a feeling of relief by all who knew her and had provided care for her. Also to their relief, the death occurred on another ward (the Intensive Care Unit), among personnel none of whom knew of her past trajectory and career in the hospital. The ICU staff confronted only a post-operative patient who never regained consciousness.

The responses of the several people who knew Mrs. Abel spell out some elements of the story of her disintegrating relationship with staff during four months of hospitalization before death. The nursing staff's great relief—the feeling that "a millstone had been removed from everyone's neck"—climaxed having been required to give comfort-care and pain medication to a lingering patient whom they could not tolerate because of her efforts to control the medication and her constant complaining and weeping for attention. The staff's concern over the pathology report on causes of her death indicated their guilt over wishing to get rid of her—a wish that drove them to the point of not speaking out against the neurosurgegry which they felt she was in no condition to survive.

The patient's doctor was concerned about the pathology report for the same reason—why did she not survive—plus the fact that he had certified the patient was ready for surgery without making a necessary test that might have indicated she was in no condition for it. The doctor's relief was also due to his getting the nursing staff and social worker "off his back" about discharging the patient for care elsewhere. He had, up to the last, steadfastly avoided this. He, too, grew intolerant of the patient towards the end—to the point of virtually complete avoidance—yet he remained reluctant to discharge her.

The social worker's relief came from no longer being forced into playing middleman between the nursing staff and the doctor in trying to negotiate the patient's discharge. Under the constant pressure from the nursing staff, she tried to negotiate a discharge that the doctor would find acceptable regarding the future care and financial position of the patient. She had found such an adequate place and public funds to support the patient, but the doctor still balked.

The chaplain's relief came from achieving closure to a case that was less than successful as he sought vainly to prepare the patient for her death. He and she never once really "communicated." At the end, he even prayed for her death on the table, "if she was going to go anyway." Near the end, he had turned her over to a theological student for practice, because of his frustration in coping with her. The husband, completely relieved, simply consented to an autopsy and disappeared.

Relief was not the only outcome of this death, for the student nurse who had cared for the patient realized that she, too, could no longer stand the patient at the end, although she had tolerated the patient much longer than the nursing staff. Despite her promise, the student nurse failed to arrive and comfort her patient the evening before surgery. For this student, however, the story was not closed with the death because of the great question it raised.

What had been the nature of the patient's dying trajectory, and the hospital career provided for it that had brought about such a conclusion to her life and such grounds for relief among the people who took care of her? The following case history of the trajectory (recorded by the student and another nurse who had done research involving Mrs. Abel) attempts to recapitulate the events that preceded Mrs. Abel's death. In the next two chapters they discuss how the nursing staff and doctor managed her pain and her last weeks and days in the hospital. The account is organized principally around the chronological ordering of the field notes taken by the two student nurses, although that chronology will be broken repeatedly for reasons discussed in Chapter I.

CHAPTER III

THE PAIN

This chapter of Mrs. Abel's case covers her initial stay at the hospital and the first weeks of her second and last hospitalization. During all those weeks, Mrs. Abel is enormously preoccupied with her pain, reacting to it in such ways that the nursing staff in turn reacts strongly against her, finding her bothersome at first, then troublesome, then "impossible." From those reactions follow a host of consequences: consequences for the nurses themselves, for their relationship with her physician, and of course for the evolving relationships between them and Mrs. Abel. This phase of Mrs. Abel's trajectory ends approximately when the nurses finally realize that she is dying —and will die on their ward. This segment of the case history, dominated by pain and its consequences, will be analyzed in a theoretical commentary after the narrative events are recounted.

STORY: THE PAIN

SA: When I started in September to study pain, I asked the nurses to describe patients on the floor who had pain. They mentioned several. Among those whom I went to see was Mrs. Abel. She was about 54 years of age and had had radiation for metastasis of the breast. She had an enlarged endematous right arm and bandaged chest. She cried frequently. When I went to see her, she explained about being in the hospital and gave some of her personal history, even about her girlhood. She brought out a picture of herself as a young woman—I guess when she was in her early twenties—with long curls. She was then a very beautiful woman. She wanted me to see how lovely she was. But she was now deformed for she had had polio as a child. Also, she told me she had had a very close relationship with her father.

She described her first husband whom she had believed would help set her up in practice as an artist. This plan had not gone very well, and she hadn't been able to follow her art career after marriage. Her second husband, whom she is now married to, is a salesman. Sometimes his business is good, sometimes it is poor. At the moment they were having financial problems, as they had just bought a new home. He had gone to Japan with a friend and had lost money in a sales transaction.

SY: There was a financial set-back prior to this illness. I might add that she had a bilateral congenital dislocated hip.

33

SA: There are no children from either marriage. She had been taking care of her mother for a long period of time just before her own illness and had actually nursed her through a final illness. Now there was no one left other than her husband.

Mrs. Abel spent quite a bit of time weeping off and on, telling about these things. Also she said the nurses didn't come in to see her very often: she frequently put on her buzzer, but no one would come. When I went out to have the nurses tell me about this patient, they told me she kept a notebook: everytime she had medication, she would jot down in her notebook what she had had—the kind of medication, the timing, and whether it was an injection or pill. She was getting both. At that time she was on methadone, percodan, and darvon. She would alternate them. She had a schedule she regulated so as to get something every hour for pain. When one nurse told me this, I realized she was rather annoyed about this. There were frequent notes in the cardex in these first two or three weeks about Mrs. Abel wanting her pain medications around the clock. Finally Dr. Colp wrote orders that she could have the medications. But the nurses didn't want to wake her up at night. Then Mrs. Abel got to setting an alarm clock so she could wake up to receive pain medication. This, of course, never goes over very well with a group of nurses who feel you should not wake up patients to give pain medication: if they're sleeping through all this, then they don't have pain! Mrs. Abel's explanation was that if she waited until morning to get the medication, the pain got such a start that the medication then didn't take care of the pain. She wanted a consistent dosage of medication; she was very frightened of pain. The nurses said the first thing in the morning—6:30—Mrs. Abel was on the buzzer for her medication. This was a real problem to them. They were annoyed, they were irritated, and they were complaining among themselves.

This had been her first admission prior to her final admission. She'd been here about three weeks. But she had been in and out of the clinic associated with the cancer ward. The ward staff frequently see these patients before they come in to the ward.

AS: In other words, when you first saw her she was merely another patient who was somewhat bothersome.

SA: Yes. The nurses were irritated and annoyed, and they wanted her to stop using the notepad for writing down the medication.

SY: The head nurse apparently told her not to use this book, and it was then that Mrs. Abel began to set her alarm clock.

SA: When I went in to listen to a nurses' "team conference" report one afternoon, they were describing Mrs. Abel. They talked of another patient who was in a room with Mrs. Abel, and a nurse said, "I wonder what she thinks of Mrs. Abel?" Another said, "Well, she just sits and looks at her"—you know, as if the patient didn't know quite what to make of Mrs. Abel. One nurse said, "Well, Mrs. Abel keeps talking about suicide," so the other patient really doesn't know what to think. There was discussion as to "do you really think she's seriously considering suicide?" The nurses didn't think so. But the aide said, "I think she means it. She wouldn't even watch television or read this morning. She seems very low this morning. She is married but doesn't have any children, and she's fifty-four years of age. She's just kind of given up." This is one of the few times the aides have said anything about this patient at the meetings.

During this early two-week period, the next thing was that the nurses stated, "She is on the buzzer all the time." There was a note about this in the cardex, but the patient told me that the nurses "keep holding off." The girls described this tactic as: "We try and get her to hold off for at least two hours between medications." Mrs. Abel was trying to get them to come right on the dot when the medication was due. She was handling her medications—ordered every three hours—and arranged her schedule so that she would get it once every hour.

Also, she was complaining about a private doctor whom she had originally seen about her illness. "I went to see him, and he told me to go home and exercise my arm." She had gone to him for a lump in the breast; he had told her to go home and exercise her arm and it would go away. So she waited for about four months and went back to him—this is a man she had been going to for a long time. Then he sent her immediately to a surgeon, because the lump had continued to grow. She complained bitterly to me that he had not done a biopsy, that maybe if he had done something she would have been spared all this. If only it had been caught in time. She said, "I have an adenocarcinoma which is one of the fastest growing tumors." This is one of the first things she told me. When I first went to that floor, it was news to me that the patients there all knew they had a cancer; but she said very openly, "I have cancer, and it is one of the fastest growing kinds, but they think they can stop it with medications." She showed me at that time, too, her radiation wound lesion which had not healed. It was open and raw and irritated, ulcerated—a very ugly thing. Later on her shoulder became very painful looking, very black.

She also said she had had a whiplash injury from a car accident. She was involved in getting the lawyers to arrange for a lawsuit to get some financial renumeration. (This becomes part of our story later.)

Soon after, she went home for a week. When I talked to Dr. Colp—I talked to him the first time she was in, too—we talked about pain thresholds. I asked, "How did you determine this?" He said, "I used a No. 25 needle and she jumped. This patient has a very low threshold, and so she will need medication. I also told her she is on narcotics, hoping that she wouldn't take very much. I tend to discourage patients from taking narcotics and will tell them that I have so many patients who are in for the same problem and only two out of twenty are on narcotics. This isn't, usually, anything that is painful and therefore, I say, you should not need very much." He hoped that Mrs. Abel would stop taking medication but she didn't. This didn't even faze her.

At the same time, there was a note on the cardex to use a No. 25, a very small needle. Mrs. Abel was getting IM injections and should have had a larger needle than a 25, but they were using the smaller. She was still jumping and complaining about how much the injections hurt.

AS: Did you pick up that the nurses had some questions about how much she actually hurt?

SA: They *were* beginning to have this feeling because, normally speaking, a patient does not jump over a No. 25 needle. It's tiny enough. But certainly there was not the degree of the questioning which came later.

During this early beginning phase of her hospitalization, I really have very few notes about her. She was not mentioned much—you know—if you asked about Mrs. Abel, the staff people would say something, but she was not constantly on the tip of their tongues.

I went back to the floor on the 20th of October and discovered Mrs. Abel had been readmitted on the preceding day. The head nurse said that Mrs. Abel was still constantly complaining and "has returned because her husband cannot take care of her"; also, the doctor admitted her in spite of his turning away of others because of his diminishing budget. There seemed to be a great deal of feeling by the RN's that the doctor was in a bind. The head nurse was sort of questioning, you know, why he had readmitted this patient. This isn't usual. She also told me the patient was admitted specifically for reasons of pain.

She was still complaining, still waking, still asking the night nurse for medication throughout the night. She was still waking up at 6:30

and asking for her shot. Dr. Colp said to keep her comfortable but don't wake her up, and this was the bind—how to keep her comfortable when she was constantly complaining. The night nurse said: she sleeps all night and sets the alarm to wake herself up, and yet she wants the medication during the night. The doctor says to give the medication to her but don't wake her up. He's telling the patient one thing and he's telling us another. He's telling Mrs. Abel, "They'll keep you comfortable," and he tells us, "Don't wake her up." So this was causing real problems then.

She was also beginning to complain of drowsiness from the amount of pain medication that she was getting, and beginning to sleep most of the time. One of the things by which nurses determine the amount of pain that patients have is how much they sleep. Are they sleeping through the pain? If so, they don't have a great deal of pain, or at least are fairly comfortable at the moment. Mrs. Abel was still keeping her medications timed so that she was getting them right on the dot of the three-hour schedule. The head nurse said, "The doctor has now ordered the medication for every two hours, but we haven't told Mrs. Abel that and so she's still running on the three-hour schedule." She was on sparine and morphine at the moment. While a staff nurse was talking to me, the head nurse went to give the medication to Mrs. Abel. It's not unusual for the head nurse to give medication. Normally the staff nurse who is medication nurse for the day will do that. But the head nurse took the medication down—a shot—and the staff nurse indicated that the patient's crying down there now because Miss Lee just gave her a shot. She also told me if you talked to Mrs. Abel, just stood there and talked to her, that she would forget about needing the medication.

AS: Did she also sleep the night through without medication?

SA: Unless she set her alarm clock.

AS: You mentioned that nurses believe if the patient sleeps the night through then the pain can't be quite that bad. Did this enter into that nurse's judgment?

SA: Yes, it did, very decidedly so. On the 20th of October, I also talked to Mrs. Abel. I had her tell me something about her week at home. Her husband had some problems in giving her medication—in controlling the amount and the time when she received the medication. She had a disagreement with her husband about the amount of dosage: he had actually given her an overdose. He had gotten confused over the doctor's orders. There had been a refill of a drug order, and he got a different dosage. So this had been a real problem at home; there had been a lot of disagreement over medication.

Then she began again to complain about the RN's forcing her to space the timing of her medication. Also, "They all give injections differently"; and some nurses hurt, some give better injections. And she had begun to play one nurse against the other, and one shift against the other. She did this by complaining about one nurse to another when the latter was standing there giving medication, or by saying, "You do a better job of this." So she would try to manipulate or coerce the girls into giving her the medication. And by trying to make friends also, siding with people. She said the doctor had told her she didn't really need to worry about medication because the drug has an effect of at least six hours; but it never works that long for her, and she has to have it more frequently.

AS: Did she have great faith in her doctor, in his being able to handle the pain?

SA: Yes, she did. But she questioned whether the nurses could; she felt that they weren't giving her the medication.

AS: But the real control was in the hands of the doctor and he could, in the end, manage it?

SA: Manage the pain, that's right. She said, "I'm on three different drugs and I'm alternating them by the hour again."

The same afternoon, when the evening shift arrived, a bull session developed at the desk between the two shifts around Mrs. Abel. The evening girl said, "I just can't get along with her. I just don't get along. I never had a patient who rejected me so." She felt Mrs. Abel had very much rejected her. I think this was connected with Mrs. Abel pitting one nurse against the other, and one shift against the other. The nurse said Mrs. Abel complained about everything she did; and when she gave the injection, Mrs. Abel would say it was the worst one she had ever received. "Mrs. Abel told me she just didn't understand why some of the girls hurt and why some didn't. When I was redressing her, she finally got to me and Elaine had to go in." Elaine is the other evening nurse, so the other girl had to do the dressing because the first girl just couldn't take it any longer.

AS: There was no indication that she had been inept, less competent than the other nurses in giving the injection?

SA: No, I don't really think she was. I would say both nurses are competent in nursing skill. As a matter of fact, the whole staff on the floor is exceedingly good. I would say rather that Mrs. Abel was playing one against the other.

The nurse also said Mrs. Abel is still complaining to the doctor that they're still using too large a needle, even when they're all using a No. 25. So now he's written an order that they have to use a No. 25.

AS: We know that Mrs. Abel is negotiating very hard with the doctor.

SA: That's right. It was Fran, the night nurse, who was talking to me. She mentioned again the bind they all felt they were in—which the doctor was putting them in—and he was in one himself with his relationship with the patient: the patient trusting him, telling the patient one thing (he could manage the pain, he could control it), and telling the nurses another thing (to keep the patient comfortable but don't wake her up, and so forth). Fran said, "Certainly she is in pain." There was not really much question that she was, although the staff had begun to question whether this was legitimate in terms of the amount of pain she had. But they all had the feeling that this woman was certainly in pain. "I should be able to do better," was what Fran was telling me.

During this bull-session, Elaine was saying Dr. Colp had gotten to where he was saying: you girls can't do anything right. He got to complaining the nurses couldn't even collect 24-hour urine correctly. The beginning of poor communication began, right at this point, between the nursing staff and the doctor. Until then there had been a fairly good communication between them. They had worked together for at least a half year.

Around that time, Dr. Colp complained about being called at night. "Why don't you call me earlier in the evening if you know a patient is going to need something or or other?" Dr. Colp's way of handling it was to write a whole list of medications that would cover everything Mrs. Abel might possibly need, so he would not be disturbed at night or wouldn't be called on a weekend. This was just normal habit of doing things; but this becomes much more significant later in Mrs. Abel's hospitalization.

AS: What you are describing up to this point is the unfolding of routine tactics used when patients have "normal" pain. The doctor does this, and the doctor does that; the nurses do this, and the nurses do that. The complex of tactics probably would not vary much from patient to patient, although the staff might use one specific tactic with one patient and not with another; but combinations of routines are building up around Mrs. Abel—and more now than say a week ago in her hospitalization.

SA: On October 21, the next day after Mrs. Abel's return, the head nurse told me Mrs. Abel had set her alarm clock at 4:00 a.m. in the morning. That pretty much is all the nurse had to say about it. So, although the nurses were still being frustrated, they felt they were still in control of the situation.

AS: Can you summarize where you stood at this date?

SA: You and I had just begun to look at the phenomena of legitimation of pain and manipulation by patients for medication. We were to look at Mrs. Abel as an example of these things.

AS: We said there was some ambiguity for the staff concerning their reading of the degree of her pain. There seemed to be some difference between her definition and the staff's. We were raising the question of "how do they read the signs of degree of pain."

SA: We had begun to look at a physician's viewpoint and the nurses' viewpoints.

On the 23rd, I went back up on the floor. They said Mrs. Abel did not set her alarm that night. The day shift felt if Mrs. Abel had done so, the night float would have blown her top, would have been very angry. Since she hadn't mentioned it, they were sure Mrs. Abel had slept the whole night through. I don't know if this was the first time, but that was the beginning of her not using the alarm clock.

The mood of the nurses was irritation and annoyance—with a patient who sets an alarm clock or who keeps a schedule. And they were frustrated. They were not sure what was going on. They didn't know what to anticipate; I'm not sure I would call it surprise because you run into this in varying degrees with one patient or another.

AS: Were they puzzled?

SA: No, because then she began to fall asleep more in the daytime and when she was eating.

That's the last time anybody mentioned her setting the alarm clock. She had been setting the alarm clock since the 19th, when she was originally admitted. But now she had gone from methadone and percodan up to morphine. She had begun to sleep more, and sleep through; so she stopped setting her alarm clock. That was the 23rd. She wasn't especially mentioned in ward conversation until the 28th.

During this period, she was one of many patients with problems of pain whom I was seeing. In fact, the staff was more concerned with and had a great deal of sympathy and empathy for another patient who couldn't swallow and who had a great deal of pain while eating. (Also, at this time, you and I began to understand how a patient's pattern and routine affected the whole ward's routine. We were thinking about patients who had difficulty in swallowing and eating who upset the ward's routine. This is significant in terms of later problems which Mrs. Abel ran into.)

On the 28th the nurses said Mrs. Abel was still the same. Nothing new was happening. "We were running at an even keel. Now she is getting morphine every three hours, and her last dose was at 5:45 this morning." The night nurse told me Mrs. Abel said to her she didn't mind dying because she was afraid of too much pain. She had talked about suicide to me before, but this is the first time that I began to pick up that the patient didn't mind dying so much but couldn't tolerate the pain.

Later in the afternoon I was talking to another nurse who said that Mrs. Abel is now euphoric, that it must be due to the amount of morphine she is getting. The nurse and I tried to evaluate this europhia: how much was due to organic reasons and how much to psychiatric reasons and tensions that might be within Mrs. Abel, leading to the amount of pain that she had and her reaction to pain. It was then, too, that she was put on ritalin, which is sort of a mood elevator.

(The other thing that you and I were looking at then was "stock-piling" of drugs by patients, and Mrs. Abel was an example of a patient who would ring the buzzer a few minutes before she was actually due for the medication to make sure that she got it. Also to make sure that she got it every three hours, so that she would never run out of medication and therefore experience pain.)

Most nurses had seen me around the hospital before this in the capacity of a graduate student nurse. Also they were interacting with me as a beginning researcher for the first time. So they played two roles with me. Part of the time I was in uniform, and the other in lab coat or in street clothes. So off and on again we switched between two roles.

On the 28th, Elaine and I were talking to Dr. Colp about sending Mrs. Abel home and about the possibility of teaching her to give her own injections so she could go home. She was requiring so much medication that a nurse would have to be there 24 hours a day. Mrs. Abel's finances wouldn't quite allow this. This was the beginning of the problem of what were they going to do with Mrs. Abel, and how they were going to get her home? This was nine days after her re-hospitalization. The nurse was concerned: at that time they hadn't tried teaching Mrs. Abel yet to give her own medication, but she felt Mrs. Abel had the capacity—partly because Mrs. Abel had given medication to her mother during the lady's last illness. But the nurses were a little concerned about the possibility of an overdose of medication.

AS: The nurses had given up on the husband already.

SA: That's right. In fact, I hadn't seen the husband yet. But he's a traveling salesman.

My feeling about Mrs. Abel's self-medication was probably pretty similar. I felt she had, probably, the capacity to learn and to give herself injections. I, too, had wondered about whether she would give herself an overdose since she had expressed the desire for suicide. I was aware of her desire to hurry the process of dying. She knew she might eventually become terminal.

AS: Did you bring this up with Elaine or the doctor?

SA: No. They were thinking in terms of over-medication and overdose, but not the full picture. They didn't really start looking at this until quite a bit later. I went back a few days later. As it turned out, Mrs. Abel was not able to give herself the injections. Since her right arm was so edematous, she could not manage a syringe to give herself the injection. This put them in a final bind because she simply couldn't give herself medication, and she was not getting any relief fr)m anything oral.

AS: If she were left handed, would they have sent her home?

SA: I question it because I had already begun to pick up the feeling of the physician, as had the nurses, that he didn't want to send her home. A couple of days later, I actually talked to him about what on earth he was going to do. But I already began to get this feeling, and the nurses began to get this feeling. This was why they were feeling the *bind*—I think. They did not actually talk about it, but the mood was there, and the feeling was there.

By this time, Mrs. Abel was on increased amounts of morphine and also on leritine, a synthetic narcotic. She could have each every two hours, alternately: morphine every two hours and leritine every two hours. So she was getting them every hour and still keeping track of everything in her book. The nurses began to say that Dr. Colp was making sure there was a whole raft of medication for the weekend, so that they wouldn't have to call him about pain medication for Mrs. Abel.

At this point June and I talked about medication. She asked what were we finding out that might begin to help them solve the problem. She felt Mrs. Abel was more afraid of pain than she was afraid of actually dying. For the nurses, the psychological aspects of death were becoming a part of the picture. Dr. Colp, as was his usual custom they felt, was side-stepping the issue and not really being honest with the patient—about her real prognosis and outcome.

They felt he was clouding the picture.

AS: Do they expect the doctors on that unit to give straight stories to the patients?

SA: They expect this, but on the other hand the philosophy is that you hold out as much hope as possible, and they are very optimistic on this whole service, so that it is sort of an ambivalent kind of expectation.

SY: In talking to the resident, Dr. Colp pointed out it's like tight-rope walking, trying to hold out hope and at the same time have the patient face reality that his life expectancy is two years.

SA: However, about then Dr. Colp told me that he was holding out hope for her but telling her that she had very little hope. Yet the nurses still felt he was really clouding the issue in making her feel that she had more to hope for. He was actually giving her a ten to twenty percent chance.

At this point I started to look at how pain may affect care, stemming from June's description to me about Mrs. Abel having to have things done in certain ways, since she was never satisfied with anything. June described: "I tried to cut her fingernails and ran into such a problem that I couldn't do *anything* right for her. It had to be done *her* way, and just *exactly* that way." June added, "I just don't know what to do with her," and was very frustrated. Mrs. Abel was on leritine and sparine around the clock, every two hours. They didn't have the alternative of choosing at night whether or not to give it to Mrs. Abel. They had to give it by order.

This dosage was contrary to the usual feeling on this floor that there is—as they say—very little pain connected with cancer. Patients are started out on gradual dosage—aspirin and so forth. Here on this floor we have a group of doctors with a particular philosophy of giving pain medication. Yet this specific patient was getting massive doses of narcotics and also sedatives. She was getting these medications on or around November 4, but she lasted for three and a half months thereafter.

The nurses were extremely busy during the month of November. There were quite a few critically ill, terminal patients then. A note on the chart said Mrs. Abel could have whatever kind of schedule she wanted for pain medication at bedtime, and by the doctor's orders she was allowed the privilege of scheduling things—to some extent. A penciled note in the nurses' planning care sheet, on the cardex, noted that the patient is very frightened about pain and keeps a schedule, and she was to be given medication every three hours. The note read, "Awake and use No. 25 needle" and also "Please awaken for meals and check her as she falls asleep during meals."

I ran in to see Mrs. Abel the night of November 4. At the same time, the nurse came in with the pills. Mrs. Abel asked if her pain medications were among the pills she was about to receive. The nurse said no, and that she would be back in about a half hour with the pain medication. I stayed about an hour and a half, but she did not mention the medication again for a while. About half an hour or forty-five minutes later she finally said, "Where's the nurse?" She hadn't realized that it had been forty-five minutes over the time she was scheduled to get the medication. I had been standing there talking about many things. As previously, she had been crying off and on.

The same evening Mrs. Abel and I got into a lengthy philosophical discussion—and this is the reason why I thought maybe she had forgotten the medication—about the meaning of reincarnation and about her religious beliefs. She had been reading some articles on the Essene.

Mrs. Abel also began to tell me about the increasing appearance of new nodules, particularly around the region of her neck, and she began to point them out to me. Her shoulder had begun to look very black and necrotic looking. There was a patient in the bed next to her, Mrs. Holt, who was also experiencing pain. She was requiring a lot of medication.

I then, on November 6, saw Dr. Colp and asked him about what he was going to do with Mrs. Abel. Was he going to send her home or was he going to keep her in the hospital? What were his plans? We were in the hallway. He spent a half hour explaining. He seemed to find a need to talk to somebody about this problem. He really was up a creek. He didn't know what he was going to do. He told me that he was going to see his supervisors and the social worker and find out what could be done, because there wasn't anyone at home to give her medication—the husband was a salesman and was away from home most of the time. When Mrs. Abel had been given insulin before, they had used an automatic injector syringe which the husband was going to bring in; and possibly, although mechanically she couldn't use her right arm very well, she could use an automatic injector type of syringe to put in the medication. He told me, "I *know* she's having pain," and that you could just look at her and see it— "all those nodules on her chest and arms." He gave a very graphic description of how horrible this was. He knew she was having pain, and he felt something had to be done. She just couldn't go home with no one to take care of her, and he didn't want to just send her to the County hospital or any place like that because nobody would take care of her there. So he wanted to keep her in this hospital. He didn't know *what* he was going to do, but he was at least going to talk to his supervisor and find out what could be arranged. He had gradually increased the sedatives and the leritine. He kept increasing the leritine rather than the morphine in order to keep her comfortable. He'd been explaining to her that the nurses couldn't wake her up to give her medication, because she still was sleeping a great deal; she had begun to sleep more and more during the day and night. He was trying to tell her "we can't wake you up to give you medication," and Mrs. Abel kept saying, "But I need the medication." So he was beginning to have problems around this issue.

The nurses were still feeling he was not aware of the basic problem. The problem was Mrs. Abel was *asking* for medication and *he* was telling *her* that they were going to keep her comfortable — but sort of ignoring that she was sleeping through the schedule yet still demanding medication and still complaining. But as we spoke, I became aware that Dr. Colp *was aware* and actually attempting to say something to the patient. The nurses were not seeing clearly what he was doing.

AS: This was the beginning of genuine animosity between the two sides. It is also the first time we really catch him in a moment of desperation, as he faces up to what he's going to do with his patient.

SA: That's right—what am I going to do with her, as she only has ten to twenty percent chance of cure? He was estimating roughly six months, in his prognosis . . . Almost a month will pass before the nurses realize Mrs. Abel is really a terminal patient though they do know her pronosis is poor.

Then we started looking at Mrs. Abel as a person who we would observe regularly. We began to predict some problems that *might* come up around her hospitalization.

At that time we thought she was going home. They were still looking for ways of getting her home, but even as Dr. Colp was telling me about this, he was planning a way of keeping her in the hospital because he couldn't see how he could send her home. Up until then we thought she might remain a week or two, or three weeks at the most, since he was using research money to keep her in the hospital *only* because her husband could not take care of her.

Then I began to focus closely on her. She was beginning to become the "patient-of-the-day" for the staff (i.e., the patient who gets the lion's share of the staff's attention). My notes become much more concerned with *Mrs. Abel.*

AS: In other words, it wasn't that you were just focusing on her in your notes. As you went around the unit, her name began to pop up everywhere when you talked with nurses. That's important to remember. It is also important to remember that we read the system wrong: we thought that it would not be able to contain Mrs. Abel for more than two or three weeks. How wrong we were! We didn't bank on research money or the anguish of a conscientious doctor. And the powerlessness of the nurses . . .

SA: . . . to be able to do anything about it. Remember, too, that we began to look at her as a patient whose whole attention was centered upon pain; the nurses' attention, too. This was the beginning of an expanding mushroom of staff focus upon the pain of one patient.

On the 8th of November, I talked again to Dr. Colp to find out what actually had transpired in the interview with his supervisor. The only way we could keep Mrs. Abel in the hospital was by making her a research patient, because the budget was getting so low they just couldn't keep her in simply because she had pain. There was no bed space, and there was no budget for her. This is the first time that he mentioned the possibility of having Dr. Tree—who was doing research around new drugs for control of pain—do research on Mrs. Abel. This would legitimate her stay in the hospital. So within two days' time, he had this arrangement made for Mrs. Abel so she could stay. He even knew what Dr. Tree was going to study with his new drug. Dr. Tree was going to compare new drugs, testing them against morphine. He would substitute his new drugs in place of morphine. Dr. Colp had tried to convince Mrs. Abel that she would stay just as comfortable with the new research drug. She had gotten very worried about the possibility of pain but took his word for it, he said. She still had a great deal of faith in him. In fact, I think she never did lose that.

He had to persuade her into this research because she was so deathly afraid the new, untested drug wouldn't keep her comfortable. But he had promised her that she would be comfortable. Also, he had to persuade her by saying: "This is the only way I can keep you in the hospital." He had no other choice. It was either make her a research patient or she had to leave. It was that simple.

But he did give guarantees that he would keep her out of pain. He said, "I kept persuading her and telling her that I would do this." I wondered at that time whether he would have to cut the medication to just percodan and the other sedative. But he said no, that they were just going to keep the medication as is.

It was the first time I had ever heard of this tactic to keep a patient in the hospital, and I began to wonder what his motivations were for keeping this patient in, because maybe other things could be done which might keep her comfortable. Did she really need to be in the hospital? And you and I had begun to recognize, first, it was pain that had first brought this lady *to* the hospital; second, pain was keeping her *in* the hospital; and third, one man now had control of *keeping* her there.

Then, too, a brief side issue came up. The nurses' notes reported the nurses had heard Mrs. Abel saying, "The doctor promised to keep me pain-free, but he hasn't." Mrs. Abel had begun to be very sleepy and to complain that she was never really pain-free in spite of the medication. Also, Dr. Colp said, "I keep her on high levels of sedation and high levels of morphine, and I'll keep increasing." He didn't know what else he was going to do, because I asked him: "What are you going to do when you reach the limits of morphine? What's happening? What can you do for this woman"? I was envisioning that he was saying to Mrs. Abel, "I'm going to keep you comfortable," while she was saying, "But he isn't keeping me comfortable now." And I thought, how much morphine can you give a patient? He began to indicate to me—this is the second time—feelings of guilt about the massive dosage of narcotics and medications that she was getting. This amount was very unusual—this much already at that point of illness. By this time he knew she was terminal, but he was still looking at her in terms of his six-months' prognosis rather than as immediately terminal. And he never was concerned with her becoming an addict.

AS: Also, you were not concerned because you thought she was terminal. We will soon see that the nurses get very much involved in the idea of narcotic addicition.

SA: Throughout the whole course of her illness her tumor growth was noticeably obvious. She was getting more nodules. They became more apparent, on the skin surface. Dr. Colp mentioned this too, in terms of legitimating her needs for medication. (Later she had increasing numbers of nodules, particularly right at the end again, so he kept changing the medication and apparently was keeping the obvious growth—which was apparent as soon as you walked in—controlled.) So now she began to have more trouble.

I began also to watch the nurses, each spelling the other. They'd walk into her room and do something or other to get the other nurse out of the room. Get them off the hook. They were getting caught in there and couldn't easily get out, so one girl would call the other girl out. She was making more and more demands, utilizing everything she could think of to keep them *in* the room. She began to take a long time swallowing her medication. In fact, a couple of times when I was there, it took a half hour. Mrs. Abel began to use methods to manipulate the nurses so that they would stay in the room. The nurses really began to be unable to tolerate her.

They were saying that they couldn't stand to take care of her because she needed to do certain things in a patterned way, ritualistically. They couldn't tolerate her—as Fran mentioned, she couldn't tolerate Mrs. Abel and had asked June to take over. And June had said, "We can't tolerate working with her for more than a day at a time." They worked out a pattern of who would take care of this patient: The aide was in on it, and so forth. They assured me that they all rotated an equal amount of time, so that all would spend some time with her.

When I talked to Mrs. Abel that night (about the 10th of November), she was very depressed. She was crying a lot, and she said, "I've been out of bed since 9:30 this morning." The nurses had gotten her out of bed and taken her down to the window. This was when they started the tactic of getting her out of her room and down to the view window—they'd take her out and she'd sit there all day long. She was still getting out and in bed fairly well by herself, but the tactic provided more things for her to watch: they were hoping that she would focus less on her pain.

About now Mrs. Abel really began to say that she was not being kept comfortable, that she was never out of pain. Most of the pain was during the day; she didn't complain much of staying awake at night. The sedatives were keeping her fairly comfortable at night. She began to describe this pain as a tight, drawing sensation, mostly in the right arm which was very edematous. She began to say, "I don't want to live. The few moments I'm free of pain aren't worth living for."

The nurses were feeling that this patient was demanding more attention and more medication than she probably needed—because she slept a great deal of the time, even sleeping through meals. She'd sleep down at the window, and the girls had already begun to feel they couldn't tolerate her, and Mrs. Abel was not legitimating her pain completely. They knew she had some pain—they all say this—but the amount was doubtful.

The girls would often be in Mrs. Brands' room. She was a very severe and critical patient, a highly valued patient, a young, beautiful Italian woman with children. I noted that the staff was spending more time and help, even more than they normally would with a highly valued patient, to legitimate staying *away* from Mrs. Abel.

The doctor knew she was terminal but was not yet accepting it. We were predicting they would either have to keep her happy or comfortable; and were already beginning to predict they were going to be unable to do either.

In reviewing my notes again, I have realized certain changes occurred over the months. Mrs. Abel in September began to tell me about her husband and some of her family problems and how she had gotten into the hospital. By November she had completely stopped talking about that and began focusing on "how large my arm is, how much pain I have, and the increasing number of nodules" that were becoming apparent. After that, she strictly focused on pain, that they were unable to keep the pain in control.

We had been talking about the period around the 14th of November when Mrs. Abel wanted to be pain-free. But she didn't want to be snowed or so sleepy and had asked Dr. Colp to cut out or at least decrease the sedation that she was getting. I think he decreased the phenobarb. I began to think about the phenomenon of a patient being able to tolerate a certain amount of pain in order to be awake. A patient would tolerate so much for something she valued.

The nurses had varying feelings about her. They described how part of the time she was tolerable, and part she was not. They were still rotating her care. The aides were supposed to be rotating one day at a time: an aide would take her during the day, and one of the nurses on another day. They could tolerate her for one day at a time. The evening girls were having more problems, probably because there were only two evening girls on, and therefore they couldn't rotate as frequently. They began to have mixed feelings about her too. Mrs. Abel was complaining very bitterly about the staff. One day she was crying and complaining that on the preceding night although she was supposed to be getting medication every three or four hours, she hadn't gotten it even though she had repeatedly asked for it. In the report, it came out, the night nurse had gone back to check but Mrs. Abel was asleep, so the nurse hadn't given the medication to her. But the next morning Mrs. Abel was complaining that they weren't giving her the medication.

Dr. Tree, by the way, supposedly had come into the picture but had not appeared. In fact, he hadn't appeared after almost a week and a half. There was never any clearcut reason as to why he didn't appear, and he had never met the patient, so I don't know what the problem was. We never did find out why he had delayed.

The nurses on the floor said they were expecting him to come about a week and a half late, but varying people were expecting him momentarily, and Dr. Colp did not know why he was late.

Since they were in the process of rotating, I talked to the aide about Mrs. Abel. I don't think the aide was as much involved really as the nurses were—although she did say they don't like to have her crying, and they were bothered by this. She said Mrs. Abel always cried, in order to get procedures done the way she wanted them done. She also described how she had to give Mrs. Abel's bath exactly the same way every day. This bothered her. She said, "It isn't as if I didn't know how to give a bath." (It has just occurred to me that maybe the reason why the aides weren't so involved is that they didn't have to fuss around with the pain medication; they weren't involved in the responsibility of giving or not giving the medication.)

On about the 17th Mrs. Abel said that now she was asking for pain medication about ten or fifteen minutes ahead of the time she was actually supposed to receive medication. It took the nurses that long to get there, she said. And she wanted to make sure that the medication actually was *there* on the appointed hour, so she would ask *at least* ten to fifteen minutes ahead of time. She would begin to put the buzzer on for the nurses, to remind them just in case they had forgotten. They were then supposed to be giving it every three or four hours—it was not a "prn" order. They were actually supposed to be giving it. She said, "I like to give them advance warning."

This was actually written for every three hours. I think by then the physician had changed to morphine, and the order was written for every three hours. "Prn," I think, at night, but an automatic order for the day time.

AS: The addiction question had not yet come up.

SA: Not for the nurses. The nurses never really talked about this.

On the 17th, Mrs. Abel was on 15 mm of morphine every three hours and was on percodan "prn." Helen said then that Mrs. Abel had put herself on a one and a half hour schedule, so that every hour and a half she got something or other. (You and I began to look at whether this is the area of contest that could occur between a patient and a nurse over the routine, and *who* was going to set up the routine at that point.) Helen was still complaining that Dr. Colp was telling the patient one thing and telling the nurses another about how much medication she could get and how often. And so Helen said, "We've sort of given up, we give her anything she wants."

Now the patient is setting the pace and not the nurses. They've given up arguing with her, are now following her routine, and she's pacing her own medication.

AS: On the cancer unit the patients often set the pace when it comes to deciding what to eat, when to take a bath, when to have their temperatures taken. But this patient is also setting the medication routines.

SA: Now on the 18th of November, Dr. Tree started doing his research with Mrs. Abel. This was when the nurses really began to really question whether she was responding realistically to pain. They always had been giving her IM injections with a No. 25 needle; but Dr. Tree was giving injections with a No. 22, which is the normal procedure. The girls said, "I don't understand how he can get away with it. She wouldn't ever let us do it." They began to question Mrs. Abel's tolerance to pain by using some objective facts. Dr. Tree was giving her the medication, increasing the amount of research drug and comparing that to the response of morphine and the response she was getting. He was also using placebos. On the day when I was there, he used the placebo without telling her. She thought she was getting the research drug. However, this followed his use of the research drug about three hours prior, and so there was some question about whether he could interpret whether his research drug was still having a lasting effect, or whether she really did not have the pain, I mean whether the placebo drug reacted the same as the research drug did. When I talked to him about a week later, he felt that she actually had pain, but that he really hadn't been able to evaluate this too clearly—other than by way of her blood pressure drop and in pupillary reaction, and there were some differences in changes. But he felt he could say she had given a good response to his drug.

I spent half an hour standing with him and his assistant at the bedside watching her reaction and watching Mrs. Abel's reaction to him. Her mood swings were alternating. She would cry one minute and then ask to have the window either open or closed, or talk about how awful her condition was and how much pain she was in. She was using the same tactics on him that she had on the nurses. He listened to her, but from my vantage point, he was listening with one ear open and one ear closed—so to speak. He heard what she said but he really wasn't listening to her. He spent a half an hour in there and then left his assistant to spend the other half hour with her. When talking to Dr. Colp and me immediately after, he said, "I just can't stand a whole hour with her." He said, "I leave my poor assistant." So that *he* also pulls out! He made no attempt to reach her psychologically or assuage anxiety. He was strictly focused on how one research drug compared with the large dosages of morphine she was on. Although he planned to do further work with her later, he never did.

AS: Did her talking get in the way of his own research observation? Did she drive him out of the room so that he could not spend the other half hour in further observation?

SA: (laughing) He just literally left. They were watching, not so much her reaction—emotionally—but her blood pressure. The assistant followed through on that. The only way, Dr. Tree said, you could really interpret whether she had pain was the amount of emotional response that she had. And, of course, with Mrs. Abel this was almost impossible to assess.

AS: It sounds like the research doctor was having essentially the same trouble, although on a more technical level, that everybody else was having when trying to decide how much pain she really did experience.

SA: That's right.

AS: It's as if everybody was saying, "She's having pain, but we don't know how much"!

SA: That's true, they didn't ever know. The common lay perspective that everybody uses involves the idea of tolerance—how much people can stand in relationship to pain. Talk to anybody and they'll tell you that some people can tolerate more than other people can tolerate or that people react and behave differently to an identical amount of pain.

AS: Would you say that running through the confusion as to how much pain Mrs. Abel could stand was the assumption that "it's hard to tell exactly what her tolerance is"?

SA: Yes, that's right, but the nurses did not use the word "tolerance" for her. The chaplain did. They never really talked about her in terms of how much pain she had. They just didn't know how much pain she had but said that she complains constantly.

AS: Yet we have heard nurses talking about this with regard to other patients: how much they could take?

SA: That's right, but not in terms of Mrs. Abel. It's not in the notes *any* place.

SY: That's true, I have not heard the nurses talk about tolerance of pain. Not in relation to Mrs. Abel.

SA: In the middle of November, Elaine was complaining about the nurses' inability to tolerate Mrs. Abel, and the rotation of people going in to answer her light. They even took turns answering her light, then. "My turn, your turn," kind of thing, you know. Then they actually had a team conference. The girls got to discussing their inability to tolerate Mrs. Abel and that she always irritated them so much that when they walked out of the room, they took it out on the next person, whoever it might be: the aide, the other nurse, or what have you. So they finally got a team conference to discuss this situation because they were all getting mad at one another since they couldn't openly get mad at Mrs. Abel.

AS: Did the nurses feel that the team conference helped?

SA: Yes, in terms of their own inter-relationships. In fact, although there was a breakdown in communication between them and Dr. Colp, there was no real breakdown among the nurses themselves. You started the next week, Shizu, and by then Dr. Colp was really pulling out of the situation. The communication between him and the nurses *really* stopped then.

I think the actual final break came when he just would not dismiss Mrs. Abel from the hospital. That was in December. The nurses got to the point where they asked the supervisor to get rid of Mrs. Abel, but the physician said, "No." That was just prior to Christmas vacation, when I took the message back to Elaine that Dr. Colp was going to keep Mrs. Abel in. But the real break came over with their getting the supervisor "in" on the situation.

AS: Had the patient now become what we ourselves call "the patient of the year" or "the patient of the month"? That is, whether day by day she preoccupied the staff members, providing the major talk and gossip among them?

SA: She had: almost all my notes are completely about Mrs. Abel. This started about the beginning of November, in spite of the fact that Mrs. Brands, who was a terminal and very highly valued patient, lay dying in the middle of December. Also Mrs. Holt and another patient died. So there were three deaths on the floor, but Mrs. Abel preempted my notes!

AS: Even the highly valued patient got less ward conversation?

SA: They were spending *time* with Mrs. Brands. In fact, they involved me in her patient care. I was in street clothes one night, taking care of Mrs. Brands. There was also a staff nurse on the floor at that time—and she spent all of *her* time with Mrs. Brands, too. Although she indicated that she felt Mrs. Abel was a patient who if she couldn't tolerate death and talk about death ought to be snowed. She was the new night nurse.

It was in the same conversation that I had with Elaine that she began to look at how miserable things were for both the evening and night nurses. Elaine then was the assistant head nurse. One head nurse had left about the first of November and another had come in, Mrs. Twist. The girls had forgotten to tell me this, but Elaine was now the full assistant head nurse who had replaced the one who left around November 1. Elaine later, in fact still, is really running the floor.

AS: When the new head nurse came in did you see any impact on the relations with Mrs. Abel right away?

SA: No, I didn't. It was in reverse: Mrs. Abel had an impact on the staff. I had a hard time setting up a relationship with the new head nurse. In fact, I really had none, although I told her who I was and she was familiar with Mrs. Abel, and we were all heavily involved in working with Mrs. Abel. (This was about the beginning of when the girls couldn't tolerate *me, too.*) I just never seemed to be there when Mrs. Twist was on the floor and never really talked with her. So I always talked to Elaine. Elaine was not only my main informant among the nurses, but she was also essentially running the floor at the time. The supervisor first begin to appear near the beginning of the year. I talked to her *after* Christmas—there were two or three supervisors ill at one time and so there was a lot of confusion in the administrative staff. She didn't get to the floor too often, but told me she'd like to spend time with Shizu talking about the care of Mrs. Abel. Toward the end of December she tried to spend some time with Mrs. Abel.

AS: Tell me about the nurses beginning to pull away from you.

SA: By and large, I talked to Elaine and June. Helen was off for a little while. I usually could talk to Helen, but I could catch Elaine and June sort of on the sly. They were still talking to me. Previously June had spent quite a bit of time talking to me about "what can we do for this patient?" But also they were really ventilating their frustrations; they're no longer asking "what can we do?" By the beginning of December, they would make a brief comment to me and suddenly get very busy with medications, or go off down the hallway, or some other place, so that even *they* began to pull out. But I have the notes from Helen, Elaine, and June about their frustrations, and they just couldn't tolerate . . .

AS: We might note here that June is a graduate of a university school of nursing. I interviewed her within four months after she'd arrived on this unit (about two and a half years ago). She was then struggling with how to handle dying patients—by herself since nobody had given her any real techniques for doing so. Then about a year ago, she was on a panel of experienced people that the Nursing Service set up, talking about the handling of dying patients.

SA: Really? And she's the one who sat down and talked to me in terms of "what can we do" for Mrs. Abel—the psychological care of Mrs. Abel.

AS: She's aware of this as an issue even though she's never really succeeded in answering it.

SA: Well, to continue: Elaine was talking in November of her complaints about Dr. Colp and the misery that all the nurses were going through, and the anticipated misery that was going to develop for them because of the research study. They did not know quite how Mrs. Abel was going to relate to Dr. Tree. They didn't know enough about the research project that he was on, but neither did I, then, to know whether this was going to affect Mrs. Abel's routine schedule. And wouldn't the research pull her off some of her medications? Would she, therefore, become more complaining, more weepy, and so forth? Was this drug going to be as effective as morphine or wasn't it? If it wasn't, Mrs. Abel was going to be in real trouble and would cause many more problems for the nurses. Elaine said, "Next week it's going to be awful for the patient *and* for *us*." The emphasis was on *us,* and "we" are going to get her constant complaints.

AS: Had they tried to talk to Colp to find out the nature of the research?

SA: No.

AS: Could he have told them?

SA: He knew that a drug was to be used instead of morphine but that all the other drugs used on Mrs. Abel would remain the same. But he didn't really know how this research was to be carried out. I had to go see Dr. Tree to find out myself.

AS: Could even Dr. Tree have told the nurses what would be the effect of their own tasks of his research? Was there any way of knowing then?

SA: Not at that point. I don't think they had done much similar research. In fact, that drug had not been used here before. This was the first patient he had used it on. When he pulled out later, he wanted to use it with a patient who had never been on the *amount* of morphine that Mrs. Abel had: he was looking for patients with fewer problems.

AS: Even if there had been adequate information between him and the nurses, it would still be very difficult to predict Mrs. Abel's reactions.

SA: That's right. He wasn't sure. But *he* was very difficult to find! In fact, I made several trips to his office, and since Dr. Colp and he didn't seem to have much communication, I became the person who had most of the information. The staff nurses were picking up information from me about what was going to happen . . . This was around the 18th of November . . .

I think I mentioned before that Mrs. Abel had mood swings. When I was there, she complained about the pills that now were due but she hadn't gotten them—and with the next breath asked the nurse who had come in to water the plant. The nurse started to water the plant with water from the pitcher, and Mrs. Abel said, "Heavens no, not with ice water." It was as if she said: "Even *I* know that you don't water the plants with ice water." So she went from one thing to another, complaining about how much pain she had and then she worried about her plant. I think this is where the nurses started to question, "How much pain does Mrs. Abel really have?" Of course, when the affair with the placebo began (and *they* were supposed to make descriptive notes that Dr. Tree could use as a reference for his research, which meant that the girls had now to spend much time in Mrs. Abel's room), then they really began to question the amount of pain that Mrs. Abel actually had.

On this same day I spoke with friends who came to see Mrs. Abel. It's interesting that only once that I know of did a friend come. I saw the husband at least two times, a friend only once. She was a next-door neighbor. Although Mrs. Abel had been crying and complaining about her arm, the friend said to me: "This is the first time that Mrs. Abel has been willing to show her arm; before she has always hidden it and thought it was a disgraceful kind of thing." Mrs. Abel was happier *in* the hospital, than at home, according to the friend. I think it was because she was getting more attention in the hospital; and also because of problems at home. That Mrs. Abel and her husband did not get along together was apparently common knowledge in the neighborhood. There had been a lot of fighting and feuding over pain, and so forth.

As Mrs. Abel's edema became worse, the right hand got puffier and puffier, and she couldn't even straighten her hand. She would say, 'Do you think I'll ever be able to straighten my fingers out again?" Her arm looked as if it was ready to split the skin, it was so edematous. She would focus on her inability to use it, along with the amount of pain, and the heaviness, the weightiness, of her arm. So I began to notice how localization of a particular body part should so engulf her attention that virtually her total life was focused around it.

56

AS: So what she was doing openly and publicly was to draw people into an orbit that circled around this particular body part.

SA: Yes. My note of November 8 says that it showed, even at this date. Although the nurses couldn't tolerate Mrs. Abel, the aide said, "She's in a lot of pain, poor thing." So the aide stuck with her at least up to then.

During Dr. Tree's research, Mrs. Abel was beginning to complain about the tension building up: "I just have to cry." She began to talk about crying as a way of relief from pain. I remember the nurses talking about how *they* began focusing on the pain, too. In fact, June said, "With some people, crying helps, but with Mrs. Abel it doesn't." But it was Mrs. Abel's feeling that crying actually relieved her tension, pain, and the whole frustration that she had built up. She said, "It's within my chest," where her lesion was anyway.

When June said this, she had a great deal of feeling in her voice, because she had begun to tell Mrs. Abel to stop crying. The nurses began to change: instead of tolerating Mrs. Abel's crying, all of a sudden they were beginning to be very aggressive toward her. "Look, crying just doesn't help you, so stop it"! It is unusual for a nurse to stop a patient in this fashion from reacting.

AS: What was their justification for this pure invasion of a patient's privacy.

SA: Feeling that they were more helpful if they became authoritarian, and very openly so. There was an interchange between June and Elaine and between June and me, particularly in terms of: we just *have* to make her do things and become very authoritarian. June wasn't using the word "authoritarian" really; what *did* she use . . . ? "Setting limits"—they had to set limits for this patient.

Actually, although they talked about it, they never really did set limits. In some sense they were going to set limits concerning her taking her pills, and so forth; that she had to do these things; she had to move around and get up. But they really stuck with her pattern. They had become used to her routine ritual and did realize that they were sticking with it. But they always talked about how it would be better for Mrs. Abel to be moved off this floor so that limits could be set. Yet Mrs. Abel had them wound around her finger, so to speak.

AS: Did they talk about stopping her crying because of her disturbing other patients?

SA: I believe this was mentioned in reference to one night when Mrs. Abel had disturbed other patients. Somebody told her that she just had to stop this: "You're upsetting other people."

AS: Were they under pressure from other patients to intercede?

SA: No, I don't think so. Unless they were picking up some cues from the patients. Nobody expressed conversation from other patients to do something, which is what happens on other floors when patients say, "I can't stand this, move me out of here." No one ever did this about Mrs. Abel. The thing the nurses couldn't stand was that Mrs. Abel even had other patients' visitors wound around her finger to the point that one went to the Stonestown Shopping Center across town and bought some shoes for her. This was a special trip—and Mrs. Abel had her take them back to exchange them!

Mrs. Holt was her roommate during this period, but she was terminally ill and most of the time she was comatose. This was the time when Mrs. Abel would snag Marilyn, who was a special student nurse for Mrs. Holt. She talked to Marilyn and Marilyn thought, "Ah, this patient is just beginning to 'ventilate' to someone. All she needs really is some attention, and so forth." Marilyn felt that she really had accomplished something with Mrs. Abel, that Mrs. Abel had sort of unburdened, and cried, and "the whole works." But I felt this wasn't helping Mrs. Abel because she had also done this with me. She had done it with the other staff nurses too, and this is why they felt that this really was not helping the patient. She was doing it to everybody she could grab hold of.

Also, there was some kind of experimental study going on in which undergraduate students were being taught interviewing techniques, and Mrs. Abel was one of the patients interviewed.

This was something that the floor just couldn't tolerate. So many people were hearing Mrs. Abel talk about her problems, therefore she was focusing too much on problems. So they pulled out the experimental interviewing. This is also why the staff couldn't tolerate me: they thought that because of my project I was asking Mrs. Abel to talk about pain. They didn't stop to find out what I was doing, where I was or wasn't; but thought too many people were causing her to focus on pain.

AS: One question: When the girls are talking about moving in to set limits on her crying, is there a tone of desperation? What is the mood? Is it anger, is it desperation, or is it . . . ?

SA: Anger. They've *had* it up to their teeth and they're going to stop this. It's, "I did this and found it worked, and I've *had* it." In fact later, but not this particular week, June describes herself as doing something when Mrs. Abel had finally gotten to her. She called Dr. Colp one night after Mrs. Abel had pushed and pushed her. So June thought she'd better check with him about symptoms. So the next day, Mrs. Abel was not bothering any other nurses, but she was calling for June and pushing her to ask Dr. Colp for more medications. June said, "I laid the law down again. I'm not going to do it." So June had begun to set limits because she felt she *had* to or this patient would use her.

AS: Did other nurses at any time, or aides, talk in terms like, "She's using me as an agent to get something?"

SA: June is the only one that did. I don't think the other girls were even that aware of what was going on. They were mad and they were angry, but not completely aware of why. They had the beginnings of awareness, but not to the extent that June did . . . . I washed Mrs. Abel's hair, too, at this time in order to chat, to see whether—well, I had a two-fold reason: one was that Mrs. Abel's hair needed to be washed again, but they just hadn't had time to do it. So I thought, I'm spending time with Mrs. Abel anyway and this would help the girls, and also my relationship with the floor staff, if I actually assumed the function for them. A second reason was that I wanted to see how Mrs. Abel would react to me. The girls would say, "I can't even cut her fingernails without her telling me how to do it." And she complains afterward. I wanted to know if she was doing this just with nurses or with anybody. So I washed her hair, and she told me once how to do it and continued to talk to me; but even though I couldn't follow exactly what she had wanted me to do because we didn't have enough curlers and things, she never complained about how I did her hair or anything about the entire process. I had to go back the second day to finish because it was late and she didn't want to go to bed with curlers in her hair. I didn't find that I had the problem that the other nurses did. Of course, she wasn't "buying" medication from me though.

AS: Who did she see you as? Who were you to *her*?

SA: A nurse doing a study, by and large, that had no connection with *what* she got. This is just a person who came in and talked to her—at that point.

AS: If you were to summarize your feelings, as you then looked at things, can you say what you believed was going on?

SA: I was seeing both sides of the issue. I could see what Mrs. Abel was doing to get her medication, and I could see that she was having trouble getting medication. She was complaining that they never brought it, that they never came on time, that they didn't believe her about her pain. I could also appreciate the communication problems that the nursing staff was having with the physician *and* with Mrs. Abel, and its inability to tolerate these problems. I think I identified with both sides.

59

Also, this is the night that I saw her husband for the first time. He was in the room when I came in. She began to talk to me about not getting any relief from her medication, not getting her pain pills, and she began to cry. The husband *got up* and *left*. He just couldn't tolerate this. He came back in a few minutes. She had continued crying. He sat down without saying where he had gone or what was going on. He asked, "Are you having pain now?" And she very angrily said, "Yes, I told you, I'm always in pain." Almost within the next breath after that, as she waited for her pills, she reached into a box of Kleenex and pulled out a ballpoint pen—to give to me. She's crying and talking about one thing, and the next thing is: "I sent my husband to get something or other for the nurses. We decided not to give candy because you know that doesn't last very long, so he bought this ballpoint pen."

When I walked out to the desk, I said to the girls, "Mrs. Abel is giving you pens." Fran said, "Oh, yeah, I see you have the latest status symbol. I had one to start with." It was her pen that Mrs. Abel had seen, and she had thought it's so useful because the pens are blue and red, and the girls alternate between using red and blue ink for charting. So Mrs. Abel thought this was a real nice gift. Fran indicated that she already had one, therefore she didn't receive the status symbol. She was almost sarcastic and disgusted with Mrs. Abel, that Mrs. Abel would use this kind of mechanism. It was with disgust that she said "status symbol." Because the girls, well, they've just "had it" by this time.

AS: Had the girls made much reference to her husband?

SA: No. When they did they indicated that they felt sorry for him, to be married to a woman like Mrs. Abel, that having to put up with her must be pretty awful. Most who spoke of him, spoke in those terms, assuming she was like this outside the hospital too.

Fran felt Mrs. Abel was very angry at her at this point. Fran was the nurse who believed that Mrs. Abel considered her not competent to take care of her. Mrs. Abel was constantly complaining. This bothered Fran because she wanted to feel that she was a competent nurse. She said, "She's so angry with me, Mrs. Abel will probably make me swallow a pen instead of giving me one." I remember Fran's emotional tone. It was "loaded" when she said ball points were the new status symbol.

AS: Did Mrs. Abel make other nurses feel a sense of professional inadequacy, dishonor that they couldn't live up to being a nurse with her?

SA: Fran was the only one that really expressed that completely.

She did that way back, early, when Mrs. Abel was complaining about infections, and it comes up again later: that she just cannot work with Mrs. Abel, and Mrs. Abel is constantly complaining about her ability. In the next breath Fran's saying that she feels sorry for Mrs. Abel, that she wants to help her but can't seem to. "Everything I do for her is wrong." This was about the 20th of November, and Dr. Colp was saying that because of Dr. Tree's coming up, he himself could escape a little more. He said that to both Dr. Tree and me.

Mrs. Abel was not, at this point, talking about death as such. June said, "She's not focused on death." But the nurses thought that her pain was heightened by her feeling that maybe the pain was related to death. We ourselves had begun to ask the question, "Is the pain and her suspicion of death correlated?" But Mrs. Abel was more concentrated on her disfigurement.

In fact, Mrs. Abel didn't then feel that she was terminal and neither did the nurses. The doctor knew it. In some sense the nurses knew that he was going to keep her in the hospital. But he never really expresses a decision that openly.

AS: The nurses, then, expected that some research would be done on her?

SA: And that she would go home—it's that simple!

We remarked earlier that the nurses did not talk about Mrs. Abel's pain tolerence. Mrs. Abel herself says, "My pain tolerance is different than other people." And I hadn't looked at it in terms of *her* talking about tolerance. It really wasn't used around her. This is something she was talking about by herself with the common knowledge that everybody reacts differently to pain. So she said, "I just can't tolerate this much." She said this back in the middle of November. As a field worker, I was assuming that she picked it up from the nurses. But it's not until now that I realize the nurses didn't use it. Mrs. Abel wanted to know, too (she was having a lot of trouble with her pain), why couldn't the nurses give her medications earlier. You know, fifteen minutes earlier, what difference would it make. She was bargaining for more medication. June said, "She asked me for it. And I just wasn't going to give it because the three hours was not up.

AS: Did Mrs. Abel ever show a genuine comprehension of what the nurses were going through and their difficulties with timing, and so on?

SA: No. . . . She took a good half hour to take medication one night when I went in the with June. June slipped me the pills so that she could go on to her other jobs. You're not supposed to leave

61

pills at the bedside at any time with a patient, particularly if they are narcotics. She could stock-pile them. I don't think the nurses were too careful about that with Mrs. Abel, and they would leave medication at the bedside. June left knowing I was a nurse, saying, "You'll be here anyway, won't you?" I said yes. So she passed over giving the medication. Mrs. Abel was annoying her because she was spending too long taking the medication. Not until the middle of November did they actually start expressing this. Elaine was the one who told me the amount of time the patient consumed. They felt even after Shizu left that Mrs. Abel required more time. They said, "Look at the number of times we *have* to be in there, just to give her medication"! Somebody had to be in there almost every hour because Mrs. Abel had it scheduled so that at every hour she had her medication. Well, it took her a half hour to take the medication, so the medication nurse was in there a half hour of *every* hour. Then the bath would take longer than that, and Mrs. Abel stretched this out. There was very little time when Mrs. Abel did not have some member of the staff in there for legitimate reasons. There was very little time when she was actually alone.

AS: Was there ever any talk about private nurses for her?

SA: No. I asked the supervisor about the possibility. She said if worse came to worse they would have to put in a float nurse as a private duty special nurse. They began to rely on Shizu. If she had had enough money, they would have hired an around-the-clock nurse at home.

AS: But she was implicitly asking for around-the-clock nurses in the hospital.

SA: And Mrs. Abel never did consider the possibility of going home herself. In fact, Shizu, when you first came in you started working on getting her out, but you said, "She won't even talk to me about it."

SY: Of course, I was pushed into it by the social worker.

SA: Mrs. Abel never did consider going home at all. That was not even a remote possibility as far as she was concerned. At that point, *she* didn't realize that she was terminally ill either. So I don't know what. . . .

AS: Tell me more about the stockpiling of drugs, and its possibility.

SA: I talked to Dr. Colp about this: she had asked him a couple of times for an overdose. Conceivably, one of the nurses was not paying too much attention about Mrs. Abel's medication. Nor were they asking questions of her when they went in her room. They stayed a very short length of time. The pills might be left there. She could have stockpiled. If she had wanted to commit suicide, it would have been very easy for Mrs. Abel to have done so. And she knew all the the drugs she was on: she knew pill by pill, name by name. She was *asking* to die and earlier considering suicide, although she never mentioned it to me at all. There was some concern about her committing suicide. It would have been very easy for her to have done so.

SY: Was this just before she knew she was terminal?

SA: Yes. She knew the possibilities. She didn't know it was a ten to twenty percent chance, but she knew that the probabilities were poor. Dr. Colp had said that he had been telling her that, and she knew that it was a very fast growing cancer, but she kept saying, "*If* they cure me, *if* they can control this. .. . ."

AS: But she could also stockpile, then give herself additional medication?

SA: That's right.

AS: Did she ever take any extra drugs by herself illicitly?

SA: None that we were ever able to pick up. The only thing I noticed was when she came back to the hospital she brought in a large bottle of percodan which the aide picked up. Now if that was actually left at the bedside, I don't know. But she had a lot of percodan at home and had brought her supply in with her. It is conceivable that she could have stockpiled that medication at the bedside.

SY: I don't think she had stockpiled.

AS: No evidence that she ever did? Never talked about it to you?

SY: No. . . . I've gone through her things many times, and . . .

AS: The medication nurse, by the way, was a different nurse each day?

SA: Yes. The team leader is usually the medication nurse, so you see the medication nurse rotates also. On the day that you were team leader you were passing out medication. So the team leader is also Mrs. Abel's personal nurse. It was foolish to assign another nurse when you were in there all day giving Mrs. Abel medications anyway.

AS: What happens to medication for other patients when she spends all her time with Mrs. Abel?

SA: When the team leader was out of the room, the aide was there with Mrs. Abel. This was the staff's feeling about it. I'm pretty sure they were right because I was never alone in the room, and the chaplain was complaining someone was always in the room.

AS: Was there somebody in the room in *fact?*

SA: Out of necessity. By and large. After you came, Shizu, you spent the first half of the day in there, and they literally had to assign an aide to Mrs. Abel in the afternoon.

AS: What did they *do* when they were in there?

SY: They did things that she requested: going to the commode, moving the arms this way and that way, getting her a drink of water. Once you got into the room there was a steady stream of requests. There was a new request before you finished the last one. That's typical of what she did to me at the beginning. And this is what she was doing to the aides.

SA: The staff couldn't pull out altogether for two reasons. There were specific doctor's orders that somebody *had* to be there. Mrs. Abel was on massive doses of medication which would disorient her. If she started to get out of bed, she could fall and hurt herself; and since Mrs. Abel was in the process of suing for a whiplash injury, there was a possibility of a suit for negligence against the hospital. This complicated the picture, and the girls were afraid—they had to obey doctor's orders, "they had to be there," or else the bedside rails had to be up. The only alternative to that was when you'd find Mrs. Abel alone at the view window sitting up in a chair, and she simply would call if she wanted something. I frequently found her here, and she would be sound asleep in a chair. If she was down there, she was by herself. But if she was in her room, usually there was someone in there.

SY: I wondered when I read in the chart that the nurse had to be there when Mrs. Abel was sitting up; I had the feeling that the doctor did not feel the patient was so bad. He was bargaining to keep the nurses in there. This is the way I read it the first time I read it, I don't know if this is true.

SA: I think this is true because he felt they were pulling out and away from her, and he wanted them to spend more time with her. Of course, it is interesting that at the end he is saying "I feel sorry for the nurses, they had to put up with much more than I did." But earlier he was really putting them in a bind by his instructions.

AS: This constant stream of requests by Mrs. Abel during this period—before the 1st of December—is there any way of telling why she's doing this?

SY: When I first met her, I thought she was so scared that this was one way of keeping people around. It's a means of controlling the environment, I thought. I still believe this.

AS: Did Mrs. Abel then know that a nurse or somebody should always be in the room with her? Was she aware of the doctor's orders?

SA: No, not then.

SY: Let's see, no. She brings it up later.

SA: She brings it up later because the staff tells her, "You can't get out of bed without one of us here." She's *aware* of that aspect of it. But she's never aware that he actually told them they have to be there as a specific order.

AS: Does she *ever* know it?

SA: No. She knows that somebody has to be there or she can't get out of bed. But she said, "I don't know what's going on because the evening girl doesn't come, the day girls do and they won't let me do anything, but the evening girls say it's all right for me to get up." This was the evening girls' response because they couldn't be there that much.

SY: She *fell*, that's the reason why.

SA: Yes, that's how she came on to it later.

AS: It's important to know that the patient never really knew the nature of the assignment.

SA: We have notes pertaining to November 22—the day President Kennedy died. I saw Mrs. Abel that afternoon. Of course, I was not in any mood to talk, so I went down to the window and sat with her. She spent an hour telling me how heavy magazines had become because people are putting in so many advertisements. "Look, if they take all these advertisings out, then these magazines wouldn't be so heavy, then maybe I could hold on to it. It's too heavy for me to hold onto because my right arm simply can't hold this much weight." She knew the president was dead and that Mrs. Hall, the patient next to her, had died that same morning. She commented, "What's the point of life, and if you've got to have so much pain then why can't you just die?" She really saw all this in terms of herself.

She had begun to get so much medication that she had gotten nauseated and was unable to eat very much. There was no real encouragement by the nurses to get her to eat. Interestingly enough, in spite of the nausea, the one time I found Mrs. Abel very cheerful was one afternoon when she was sitting at the window. This was one of the few times that I actually saw her that *I* could describe as cheerful. In fact, it's the only time, come to think of it. I guess this was because she had gotten so much medication that she was kind of euphoric. Later they had to cut down on it. She was then on 20 mg of morphine.

Miss Wilson, the new night nurse whom I spoke to that same day, gave the first indication that some nurses would possibly "snow" a patient, to a certain degree, but that they wouldn't push it past the respiration point. Where respiration was so depressed that the patient might die, they might give as much medication to keep them comfortable as they felt they could.

My next notes on Mrs. Abel simply say that she was the same. I remember that there was nothing really new during this time, and no great changes apropos of Mrs. Abel. It's then that Shizu starts working with her.

AS: This period of time covers what dates?

SA: My notes are between November 22; and then I skip down to the 2nd of December when the next big change occurs.

AS: We should now turn to Shizu.

SY: For about a week prior to taking care of Mrs. Abel, I began to hear an awful lot about her, in reports, in careful conversation—mostly griping about Mrs. Abel. A great deal was in terms of the problems they were running into, and the giving of narcotics to Mrs. Abel. I kept hearing over and over again that she wanted to be awakened at night for her medications. The "rand card" at that time said, "Do not awaken for medication." On November 26, I was in a position to pick a new patient to take care of. What I had been interested in for the past month and a half on the cancer unit was how better to relate to dying patients: so I had been taking care of patients who have not been responding to therapy.

AS: Did your previous patient die?

SY: No. I realized at this time that once a patient becomes terminal then he gets ignored. I had great difficulty in getting information and help from the rest of the staff concerning how to take care of the patient.

One other point that would pinpoint my feeling then: I thought I should tell the assistant head nurse what I was doing. I was interested in knowing how to relate better to dying patients and therefore I would be taking care of patients *not* responding to therapy.

SA: How did you know that Mrs. Abel was terminally ill, since the nursing staff did not then know?

SY: My assumption throughout all this was that any patient who is not responding to therapy is one who is terminal. It's just a matter of when you talk about terminality—in terms of two days or three days, you know. But *my* focus was that the patient is dying either rapidly or slowly. The patient is dying; this is my focus.

AS: How did you first begin to hear about Mrs. Abel while still nursing your other patient?

SY: I was hearing her *not* in terms of her dying, because the staff's focus then was pain. But I assumed that where the focus is on pain, and where the staff is trying to keep the patient comfortable, then actually the patient *is* in a stage of terminality—when he is no longer responding to therapy. The staff's focus is not therapy; the focus is on keeping the patient comfortable.

Before when I picked out a patient to care for, I went around the ward talking to patients. This was different. I asked the head nurse to suggest pain patients, and she suggested two patients, one of whom was Mrs. Abel. Then she described Mrs. Abel as a "lulu," meaning that she whined, cried, and was preoccupied by pain. Then when I asked if this was the patient whom 1 had been hearing a great deal about in reports and around the ward she said, "That is the patient"! Then the head nurse went on to say that this was the patient who slept through the medication at night and who insisted she be awakened.

Anyway, I went to look at the two recommended patients and interviewed them. The first interview was with Mrs. Abel. She was sitting with a very sad look on her face. Her gown was open and her bandaged breast exposed. She was a pretty horrible sight to look at, with ugly lesions, and her arms were very, very edematous. Immediately after I introduced myself, she began to tell me all about her complaints; about all the medications she was on. Then she told me how artistic she was, that she had real sensitivity toward art and this made her more sensitive to ugliness than other people. She showed me a picture of herself when she was 27 years old. She looked sweet-sixteenish.

The other interesting thing was that she opened a portion of her dressing to show me the lesion. At the same time, she did not look at me to see what kind of facial expression I myself had. Then she told me about all the drugs she was on, and described some therapy that Dr. Colp was looking forward to and that she hoped would cause a regression of cancer. Then she said she couldn't go home because of the pain and described her husband as becoming very, very upset, saying that he was a very nervous, inadequate person. She couldn't go home for this reason.

SA: Who were you to her? Did she know that you were part of the floor staff? How did you introduce yourself?

SY: I can't remember. I just introduced myself, giving my name, then "It" just poured out. The following day, though, I told her I was a student nurse. I was in a lab coat.

She made a special point that she could not go home because of the pain and because of the situation at home. Then, at the same time, she talked about the new drugs that the doctor was looking forward to trying on her. After talking to her, I felt, "I'll take a whack at caring for her." She would certainly be a challenging patient. I announced to the head nurse that I would be taking care of Mrs. Abel. She immediately wanted to know how many mornings I would be going up there, although she already knew. She said "good" because the patient was *so* impossible they had to rotate the staff around. No one could stand being with her for days on end. I became curious to find out what this patient does that makes everybody react so violently to her. This was what I was interested in, and that was what I was focused on the following morning. I sat back and . . . .

AS: Did you have secret feelings yourself that you could manage her?

SY: Yes. So I immediately began to read through the patient's chart, gathering as much information as I could about her history. After I wrote, "With her physical history, it's no wonder that she is having difficulties and is also difficult. She probably comes here with a very damaged body image and cancer probably increased this, and pain therefore would be more severe. Also, with her physical problems and her past history, she has very deep seated emotional problems, and this illness is going to make it more severe."

By the time I got to take care of Mrs. Abel there was already a clear schedule worked out for her for narcotics: first, morphine; one and a half hour later she would get sparine and percodan; and then morphine. In other words, every one and a half hours narcotics were given, and the schedule had been going on for some time. I decided that I wasn't going to fight it. I was going to follow this routine. Another thing is that the staff had been telling me that she sat with a book marking down very carefully when her narcotics were due. Mrs. Abel would turn on the light ten to fifteen minutes before the drug was due in anticipation of the drug and also of warding off the pain.

68

SA: Nurses just cannot abide people who invade the nurse's territory. "*We* are the ones who schedule medication." And to have a patient say that she is going to schedule one—and *then* to sit and write it down! That seems really to cause frustration for the nurses and they get angry.

AS: Yet they also know that patients do this frequently all over the country.

SA: Yes, but it's the one thing that will cause *any* nurse to become irritated, almost without fail, in any situation I've ever been in. . . . The other thing is that on this floor the nurses very early told me, "Cancer patients do not have pain. We have difficulty in making people from other floors understand this." Here is this patient, Mrs. Abel, who is requiring massive doses of narcotics and yet the nurses feel that there shouldn't be pain. The patients don't have the pain, but everybody on other floors think they do.

AS: That's part of the ward's ideology. The staff makes clear distinctions according to the type of disease and its progression. But they think that this particular type of disease apparently shouldn't have quite so much pain, ordinarily.

SA: That's right. However, the doctor felt this particular one is always connected with pain. The other physicians on the floor feel that you start from an aspirin and work up, except when a patient has recognized massive pain; but this particular physician feels that cancer is a disease that usually has pain. He doesn't like to use narcotics, but occasionally will.

It was on November 25, the day Shizu was coming in, that Dr. Colp pulled out—in the sense that there wasn't anything more he could do for Mrs. Abel. He did all he could. He knew there wasn't anything that was going to help her. He was going to hold her on what medication she was now on. Because when he changed drugs then her level of hope would drop noticeably. He was actually postponing the change of drugs, although he should have changed. In fact, he kept her almost a month longer. . . .

AS: He was playing a very interesting game of timing.

SA: Using her hope in medication, that's right, and the amount of morphine she was going to get.

AS: And this is all the more interesting because now Shizu comes on the scene not knowing any of this and makes the decision in terms of "well, these are the rules of the game" that she's going to play by. If she challenges them she runs into too much trouble.

69

SA: And Dr. Colp has indicated, "I have quit taking her home with me." (As a problem after hours.) He quit talking to me after this. He said, "I'm not going to take this home with me anymore; I don't want to talk about it." Consequently Shizu runs into problems with him almost immediately. And again he referred to his budget, "As soon as Dr. Tree finishes his research, I'm going to discharge her. I can't keep her in." But he changes his mind. He vacillates later.

SY: The following morning I was greeted very cheerfully by the assistant head nurse and the staff. Previously they had been pretty much ignoring me. I thought, "Well, I guess I'm in like Flynn now because I'm taking care of this 'ward pill'." When I took care of the previous patient, I had asked how they felt about giving narcotics to the patient. The medicine nurse had preferred to give them. With Mrs. Abel, I decided there was such a big fuss about medication that I offered to be responsible for the narcotics. They very gladly and very happily relinquished the job to me. The medicine nurse, at that time, said that she would appreciate this because it was so difficult to give Mrs. Abel the drugs *exactly* on time, and if you were five minutes late, Mrs. Abel would almost fall apart.

Also, on the "rand card" was a statement, "patient gets shampoo." I didn't know then who was supposed to do it, or what was involved —but I'll go into the details later. As soon as I entered the patient's room, she began to tell me all about her aches and pains. This went on for about ten minutes. She complained bitterly about not getting her injections at night, that she had to call for them, and by the time she called for the nurse the pain had really gotten a good hold of her and it took at least about an hour to overcome. She had to tell me, "I have pain *all* the time, my dear," and went into a long description of where it was and pointed to her hands, her fingers, and all. Then she pointed to her neck and pointed out that she was getting a few more nodules and said that she hoped they would not continue.

I thought that she abruptly changed the subject because she brought out a picture of herself when she was 27 years old. She looked sort of Alice in Wonderland with long pretty hair, and a long dress where the deformity of the hips was not visible. She described herself as being quite withdrawn, that she tended to live in her world of books and art, and then she talked about what beautiful hair she had at that time. She talked in great detail. I thought, well, maybe I'd better wash her hair because it was very important to her. Then she talked about this artistic ability, and I got curious about it so I let her talk. I questioned her and found out that she had really not seriously painted since the age of 19. I thought she certainly has an elaborate illusion to escape her past ugly world and the ugly world of right now.

In discussing this later in the morning with the staff I gathered that the staff kept saying, "You know she really hasn't painted since she was 19." They did not realize that this was an illusion that the patient had to maintain to face the ugly world. I was critical of the nursing staff for not picking this out, and I didn't know quite what to think. Were they at a point where they could no longer have any objectivity about Mrs. Abel?

The first days I was just going to sit back and let Mrs. Abel do all the talking. Actually that wasn't very difficult because it was just a monologue. Anyway, breakfast came up, and she began to complain about being nauseated and that nothing tasted good. So I sat by her and we talked about all kinds of other things and she ate· There was no mention of nausea for the rest of the morning. I was curious, she always started the morning off with nausea, and I let her know that I would be with her all morning long. I would stay with her for breakfast, and there would be no discussion of naseau. So I figured this was her way of getting sympathy.

I was also fascinated by the injection. I went into her room with her injection *on time*. She brought out her little book (which was carefully hand-lined). It had the time the drug was due, and on it was *right, left,* indicating which hip each injection was to be given. Then she wrote the time down in red; after the drug was given it was carefully crossed out with blue ink—because she said that previously she used to do it all with blue ink, but then she couldn't see the last time she wrote on it. I was fascinated by all of this, watching this whole thing. I thought, "Gosh what an elaborate system of controlling the environment and the means of warding off pain." I realized I was not going to argue with the book; I was going to let her write in the book, and I was going to give her the drugs exactly on time.

I did have to plan ahead of time, though, because this giving of narcotics was a major task! The medicine nurse or the head nurse usually carries the keys to the narcotics box, and each time you give her narcotics you have to get this key and sign out for it. Many times you can't find the medicine nurse or the head nurse, so if you want to give the drug exactly on time you have to plan quite a bit ahead of time. I found myself in later periods catching the nurse an hour or a half hour earlier so that I would have the drug ready. One of the rules is you don't prepare the narcotic until you are ready to give it, but this one I broke and nobody seemed to question it. So I'd have it ready, sitting there to go; or many times I would take it right to the patient's room with me and leave it there until I was ready.

SA: Did you ever use a No. 25 or a No. 22?

SY: Oh, that's another thing· It said on the nurses's "rand" that it was to be a No. 25, but I couldn't find a No. 25 once. That was the first day. I said, "You know, I can't find a No. 25 needle," and I think it was Elaine who said, "Go ahead and use what you have." So I used a No. 23. The patient did not make any noise about it at all. As a matter of fact, she said, "I wish they all gave it as nicely as you do." I kind of laughed to myself because I thought, "I'm up to your tricks, you probably do this to every nurse that comes in, you say something good about them and something bad about the past nurse·"

SA: Why didn't you question the No. 25 order?

SY: There was something on the nurses's "rand" indicating that she was very—I can't remember whether it said she has a low tolerance for pain or not. And that's the reason why I used the smaller needle.

I was fascinated by this drug keeping, this record keeping, and I asked her if this helped her in keeping an account of the drugs. She said that if she didn't keep an account, then the anticipation of pain became so great that she couldn't stand it any longer—and it took some time for the drug actually to work. Then she went on, as she did in the following days to mention a lot of things that the doctor was hoping to do, in terms of therapy, to reduce the cancer process; although at the same time she said that being kept alive was no help because one had to consider how one lived—and being kept alive was all pain and ugliness which wasn't worth it. She vacillated back and forth throughout the morning about the new drug, full of hopefulness and at the same time wanting to die.

Then I decided to shampoo the patient's hair. I asked her how to go about it. It was the kind of situation where she had to point out every step involved· You come in at that time, Shirley, to observe, and you probably noticed that she wanted it this way and that way, and was very specific about how she wanted it done.

SA: I made a notation that she was a little more particular about this routine with you than she had been with me in the preceding weeks. This is the first time I had even realized you were in the situation. It was at this point that we encountered each other—over a hair wash.

AS: And explained to each other what each was doing there.

72

SA: Yes. The next time we got together was later that afternoon. It was the 4th of December.

SY: This putting up of her hair was accompanied by detailed instruction. The problem was that I told her I wasn't very good at putting it up. This cued her that I wasn't sure, so she was going to play it for what it was worth. Then, throughout putting up the hair, there was a steady stream of conversation about when she got married and all her past life. When I would say, "Well, now, earlier you said . . ." trying to clarify some point that she had talked about earlier, she would say, "Now wait a minute, let me finish this." This pattern was to be used throughout the next weeks. I thought, "This is the way she controls everybody that comes into her room."

AS: What did pain mean to this lady as you then saw it?

SY: Pain re-emphasized the damaging of the body image, and, therefore, all of the things that she had been telling me about her artistic sense and all this sort of thing indicated to me that the pain was a representation of damage to the body image. Pain also, by the process of her record keeping, meant the controlling of the environment.

Keeping these schedules and everything helped control the environment and, at the same, time, warded off anticipated pain.

After the shampoo she had been given the usual morning routine, and I reported to the team leader. She hoped the shampoo would keep Mrs Abel happy because apparently Mrs. Abel had been pestering everybody to do the shampoo.

SA: What's intersting is that the time length between your shampoo and my shampoo was one week. The time length between my shampoo and when June shampooed her was about three weeks. So the shampoo came closer and closer together at this point of her illness, when she couldn't tolerate pain.

SY: Helen made the statement that she felt all kinds of people were talking to Mrs. Abel about pain that this was focusing the patient on pain. What she thought the patient needed was distraction. So I said, "Do you think it's possible to get Mrs. Abel to stop thinking about pain or her problems?" Helen repeated she felt that she thought it was bad to focus on pain, then added the patient wanted the heavy doses of narcotics so she wouldn't have to think about things. I thought, "How strange, she's thinking about this in two different ways."

AS: It's also very fascinating that here we are in late November, having gone through a month and a half or more, during which they literally have had their noses rubbed in her pain. They can't avoid the subject because this lady's been bringing it up again and again. Now we hear Helen saying that if only she could get this woman off the subject by focusing on something else—and as *if* the *outsiders* somehow had brought up the subject and not the lady herself. It's a desperate movement on her part for she must really know that neither the nurses nor the researchers brought this up.

SA: My notes on the 4th say that June complained that Mrs. Abel was using her and wanted to get her sympathy. The next day Mrs. Abel singled June out to get more medication and June said, "I just told her I wouldn't," and that she had all the medications she could have and that she was to stop complaining and eat. June was very angry. And Mrs. Abel did eat. So June said she was going to use that tactic again. It worked.

SY: At that time, I made a notation that everything Mrs. Abel did seemed to be on controlling the environment, and that she probably had married an inadequate man. Again, someone, she could control. She described her husband in a way that actually emasculated the poor soul.

The the following day I ran into Dr. Colp. I asked what the plan of care was, and he said that he felt nothing more could be done for her. But he was more concerned with trying to keep her free of pain. At the same time, he mentioned that he was thinking of playing around with another hormone—which I thought was very strange. He felt that he had carried Mrs. Abel as long as possible beyond what was reasonable in terms of research. Mrs. Abel's stay must be terminated. But he was "up a tree" because the only recourse open to Mrs. Abel was to go home, and he was petrified of the idea. And he could not accept the other alternative of going to the County Hospital. Also, he felt that it was not a good idea because there was a lien on the house when accepting Mrs. Abel as a patient. He described the whole situation as poor and Mr. Abel as being beat down, and that he probably would be beat down too if he had a wife like Mrs. Abel He appreciated what was happening to the husband, and he said that the awful part of it is that there is nothing you could do except to tolerate it. He went on to say, "I know. I went through an experience just like this with an immediate relative of mine, and there is nothing you can do except tolerate it." He described this relative who had the whole family in an uproar.

Then he complained that he got it from all sides—he got it from nurses and he got it from the patient. I asked if he had contacted the social worker and he stated that he had; she was looking for some place to discharge the patient. I wondered if he was running into difficulties in getting Mrs. Abel discharged because of his personal experience.

AS: Do doctors usually talk this freely and at such length to you when you nurse special patients?

SY: Yes. . . . We must have been standing twenty minutes or so. General frustration was the feeling I got, that he didn't know quite what to do, reciting his own personal experiences in similar situations, feeling badly about having to discharge her because the situation for discharge was poor.

*   *   *

AS: This is two days later, and the girls are going to report what has happened since the last time we met.

SY: I checked out some things. I talked to the night nurse who came back in the middle of November, and also a seminary student. The conversation with the night nurse was subdued compared to the conversation with other nurses. She stated the patient had the quietest night before surgery, compared to any other night that she had been on. Also, the patient only had one injection of morphine during this period, which was unheard of because it had always been every three hours. Also, Mrs. Abel was the most trying patient that she ever encountered. She thought that the patient was most agitated during the month of January. She described Mrs. Abel's awakening and screaming out, which would awaken the rest of the patients, thus creating all kinds of nursing problems with running and taking care of these awakened patients—and then running to take care of Mrs. Abel. She cited an instance when there was a patient dying across the hallway and Mrs. Abel was very upset that evening. Finally she sent in the one and only aide, that she had, to quiet Mrs. Abel down. She felt sorry for Mrs. Abel but finally she just had to learn to ignore her because she couldn't be in the patient's room. She is a young nurse. She graduated in September and came to CRI in October. This is her first job. While she was in college, she had to leave because her mother entered the terminal state from cancer of the breast, and she took care of her for several months before her death, giving the injections. Afterwards she entered a school of nursing. She compared her mother with Mrs. Abel, describing similarities and dissimilarities. The similarities were on the question of pain She, too, had to run away from the patient, not so much because she didn't want to be with the patient (that's the feeling I got) but because of the pressure of the ward. She is the only nurse on nights, plus one other aide (or maybe two aides), so she can't talk about this problem to other nurses as she could on the PM when there are two nurses or on the day shift when there would be a number of nurses.

SA: She hit nights about the 3rd of December.

SY: I should add she had the experience of the patient reaching out and crying, "I want somebody to love me." This nurse said, "I knew what was happening so I took her in my arms." I believe this nurse is the one who is most disturbed by this whole experience.

AS: You are describing a staff person who is having her own private experiences, relatively out of contact with the rest of the nursing staff. I doubt that anybody on the staff knows what has been going on with her.

SY: Yes, because I hadn't known this either when I talked to her earlier. When I started the conversation with her the other day, I knew something was going on and that I had to sit it out with her. Then she began to describe how she made the comparison of Mrs. Abel with her mother. She dwelt at some length on this.

AS: Two years ago when I interviewed June on the evening shift, when she was a young nurse six months out of college, she described how she was wrestling with the problems of handling her own feelings of death and what death meant, and she also related certain experiences she had with a patient who reminded her of her mother. What came through in her description was this sense of personal search and anguish without any communication with the head nurse or other nurses on the floor. She described staff communication about specific patients, but not communication about what she or anyone else was going through personally.

SA: When I was talking to June last night she said that the girls on the floor still can't stand to talk about Mrs. Abel. I asked whether at the end Mrs. Abel had reminisced at all. June said "no" that she only did that in the very beginning· "I guess we finally let her know that we were unimpressed and she stopped." Stopped telling her life history; how beautiful she was; her many husbands, her art life, and so forth.

Then June said, "She was ready to end the story. She had become resigned to the surgery but because it had been postponed and postponed Mrs. Abel wasn't sure whether she would die without having surgery or whether she would die on the table. Mrs. Abel knew she was dying the last couple of weeks, but she didn't go over any past history with us." Then she added, "There was no reciprocity between Mrs. Abel and the staff." She explained it by saying, "She wasn't sincere; she didn't share any feeling or any sense of appreciation." This is the same thing, Shizu, you were talking about. The girls didn't feel that Mrs. Abel "appreciated what was being done." The only times they had talked about her, by the way, is when Shizu had been on the floor—which is rather interesting. June went on to say, "When I go into a room (meaning Mrs. Abel's room which is now 'Mrs. Abel's room'), I think it is different. It isn't like it used to be when Mrs. Abel was here."

June also said that although she had been losing her temper with Mrs. Abel, it didn't help. She said this with a sad quality, not one of anger or frustration. She hadn't really been able to help Mrs. Abel no matter what she did. Even losing her temper—which she feels badly about—didn't help Mrs. Abel either.

SY: She said, "Nothing worked with her."

SA: She is looking at herself and feeling maybe I could have done more. She conveys a sense, I think, that there was something about Mrs. Abel that she should have liked. During our conversation she also noted that finally the staff had been able to have a conference and work out their own personal problems, which they hadn't been able to do until last week, when there was a change of staff· Now they are beginning to talk to one another.

AS: What happened at this meeting last week?

SA: I didn't ask. June said, "We finally were able to talk about the difficulties and changes and our personal problems and the tension that was amongst us since the change of staff." I didn't think about asking her . . .

SY: Now I will tell about Mr. Thompson, the seminary student in the chaplain's seminar. This is the gentleman whom the chaplain sent in at the very end. Mr. Thompson is a man in his forties. He has been a pastor for some seven to eight years in Los Angeles· He was assigned to Mrs. Abel by the chaplain because Mrs. Abel, at least when she was admitted, put down that she was a Methodist, and Mr. Thompson is a Methodist minister. He had seen Mrs. Abel three times, one time a week for three consecutive weeks prior to her death, and the last time was the day before surgery. He started off the interview by saying he "got to her" quite quickly, for as soon as they met she began to open up and talk about her problems. When I questioned him about the content it was pretty much the content that all of us had been exposed to on our initial encounter.

He gave the impression that everything was sort of real cozy and that they got along fine. I thought he couldn't have gotten through;

nobody else got through! I couldn't get through so he couldn't get through! He said during the second interview the patient dwelt on wanting to commit suicide and kept asking why God would permit someone to be in pain. I asked Mr. Thompson if he found this difficult to deal with. He said no, he felt fairly comfortable with this. I thought "it can't be that hunky dory," so I discussed my own frustrations in dealing with this patient and described what she had talked to me about. It was at this point he said the chaplain had told him the patient had blown off about the things she had been telling everybody else. As he listened to me talk about my frustration, he finally came out and said he was *very* uncomfortable in the last interview, and he was relieved when he left the room, which he did earlier than he usually did in previous encounters with this patient. That evening he went home and really thought about whether he really helped the patient and reevaluated his discomfort during this experience. It made him think about the things he had done in the past and whether they were really comforting to the patient.

He said it really made him think. Apparently he didn't arrive at any conclusions, but he said he really had to think about it and re-evaluate some pretty pat answers. Then I saw the chaplain shortly afterwards and he stated he had spent some time discussing Mrs· Abel with Mr. Thompson, who had found the experience with Mrs. Abel a very disturbing one and a very thought-provoking experience.

AS: It is very important for these men to get through to the patient because that is their mode of operation. They don't give care to the patients as the nurses do: the only thing they do is to get through to terminal patients and comfort them and prepare them for the transition to death. So actually the chaplain very often moves in at that stage of dying when the nurses say there is nothing more to do—it's precisely at this point that the chaplain finds there is a great deal to do and is able to do it successfully sometimes. So he is imparting this knowledge and mission to Mr. Thompson, his student. It is also interesting that Mr. Thompson is an older man who has come to a teaching center from as far away as Los Angeles in order to learn the techniques of handling patients when they are either terminal or in other acute disease phases. You would not find this at most hospitals because there are few of these except at teaching hospitals.

SY: Now let me clarify the confusion about the lien on Mrs. Abel's house. The social worker—who I have asked about the lien— stated that it took an awful lot of rigmarole to straighten out the confusion about the lien for Mrs. Abel's potential admission to the City and County Hospital. The difficulty was partly due to Mr. Abel's agitation. It was very difficult to get the facts of the situation. Also, she felt there was an almost deliberate attempt by Mrs. Abel to confuse the issue because having a lien on the house meant that she could not get into City and County—so she kind of dragged this confusion out. Anyway, the facts are that back in 1961 Mrs. Abel was hospitalized in City and County following her whiplash injuries sustained in this accident· The hospital at that time placed the lien on her house for payments of services; however, she was able to get a friend to put up a second mortgage, and in a matter of three months she had paid off the hospital bill. After the bill was paid, the lien was removed.

SA: Mrs. Abel knew that.

SY: Anyway, on the basis of this experience, Mr. Abel and Dr. Colp assumed that this is what would happen if they were to transfer her to City and County. When the social worker examined what the financial situation was, the assets and all, she found the Abels were in great debt because of the husband's financial setback. She knew that the lien from the previous experience would not be required for admission to City and County, so she checked and found that the patient would be eligible for aid to totally disabled—and this would enable Mrs. Abel to be admitted to City and County and to other available nursing homes. The interesting thing, she said, was that once the arrangements were made, Dr· Colp had to be told over and over again that this was the situation. "I had to tell him over and over again, at least twice a week after it was arranged," to ressure the doctor that a lien was not on the house.

SA: There was a lot of confusion about this and there must have been a great deal of communication between them, because one of the last times I talked to him in January he was very concerned about this money. He said that part of the problem was Mr. Abel had to have a fluctuating bank account because he was a salesman; sometimes during the month he would have as much as $1,000 in the bank and then he was no longer eligible for the aid to the totally disabled. The doctor went into a long harangue about people who have saved all of their lives shouldn't have their life savings wiped out because of illness.

SY: But the social worker was saying, "I don't know how many times I had to tell him and explain to him that actually Mr. Abel was in so much debt anyway."

AS: When did the social worker really know that she could get the maid for the needy?

SY: Early in January she stopped me and said all the arrangements were made. She can get into a nursing home, and the nursing home in Contro Costa County accepted patients in her condition because they had a lot of vacancies.

AS: Now let's get the timing straight: she finally made this arrangement, after Dr. Tree pulled out and just before the speculation about a lobotomy.

SA: I have interviewed two people today—one was Miss Lyon (the Supervisor) who was away at the time of surgery and since then for about a week. She said the girls haven't even mentioned Mrs. Abel to her.

AS: Did she herself ask about Mrs. Abel? Was she curious? Did she want to know what went on?

SY: She said she was pussyfooting around because she didn't know whether to raise the discussion or not. "They haven't talked about it." She felt that they had talked it out the first week, as the staff up there generally talks over their problems. I thought, "Good God"!

SA: She said, "I haven't noted any repercussions." I asked her if she had expected Mrs. Abel to go to surgery. "No, I expected them to postpone and postpone and postpone until they finally couldn't do anything because she was a poor surgical risk, or that she would just die before they could do this." She said, "Really I didn't expect them to do it or, if they did, I expected her to die on the table because of her poor respiration." If Mrs. Abel had lived through surgery, arrangements had been made that she would go to the 7th Floor automatically.

AS: Four years ago there was a panel consisting of a doctor, a nurse, an aide, a chaplain, and so on. The panel was on the problem of dying patients. Miss Lyon was the nurse who was selected as one who had worked with dying patients and articulate about it; indeed, she did very well. Now we see her four years later.

SY: Did she say the staff didn't have any guilt felings about Mrs. Abel?

SA: She said they hadn't mentioned her. She hasn't talked to them at all.

SY: She said to me she didn't think they had any guilt feelings. Actually they were busy with other concerns.

AS: It sounds like she has remained fairly distant from the whole sad episode from the very beginning. Or do you feel that is not true, do you think she was really in there?

80

SY: She was very concerned about the staff. This is mostly what she dwelt on.

SA: She said she spent a lot of time on the floor, but this was in January. In December she got involved in pushing Dr. Colp to get Mrs. Abel out.

SY: Miss Lyon said she was spending about ten to fifteen minutes with Mrs. Abel about every other day, just going in and talking to her and having her discuss surgery. She said there were times when she was busy and couldn't do it, but she made it a point to go in every few days. But I never did see her on the floor.

SA: My impression was that she was very involved with the staff as early as December when Elaine was pushing to get Mrs. Abel out of the hospital prior to Christmas. Miss Lyon really put the pressure on Dr. Colp at that point to get Mrs. Abel *out*.

I talked to her in January and during the Christmas holidays. There was a lot of illness on the part of the staff, and Miss Lyon wasn't on the floor about half the time. She had been away at several intervals during Mrs. Abel's hospital stay. So that's the one point I know she got involved. She told me then that she was trying to spend some time with Mrs. Abel in order to relieve the staff. But I never did see her on the floor.

SY: I ran into her on occasions, but she actually did not come in to see the patient on days that I was in the room.

AS: What is your impression of the general role of the supervisor on this kind of unit?

SA: Most supervisors do not find time to check to see about critical or terminal patients or if there are any family problems.

SY: She said she was terribly concerned about the staff and always has been more concerned with the staff on CRI than other floors because, "You know, you get to a point where the patients really get to you," and she watched for this kind of thing. She said she had tried to relieve the situation, helping whenever she could.

AS: She has been a staff nurse at this hospital, and an assistant head nurse, and a head nurse, and supervisor. She's been through all the steps, and when she talked at the panel she reported very faithfully what goes on from the point of view of nurses· So she has never been distant from the operations of the floor. But it's my general impression that the supervisor is mainly concerned with the staff, with certain kinds of fights, and that there's relative autonomy on the part of the head nurse.

SA: Yes, I think this is true, particularly on this floor—as it is on almost all floors.

SY: She said the staff up there are a good bunch of kids and they work quite well together, that it was a rough floor, but they handled the situation as best they could and did a fairly good job. She repeated this over and over again. She said she felt sorry for Dr. Colp because he couldn't get rid of Mrs. Abel. Then I asked her, "What do you think could have been done so that it wouldn't have grown to the proportion that it did?" She really didn't know; she didn't think there was any answer to this. She did feel that Dr. Colp could have lessened the tension between the two of them had he indicated to the nursing staff that Mrs. Abel was a terrible patient, and let the staff know that he appreciated what they were doing; but he did not do this until the very end and at that point it was of no value at all to the staff because they were very angry. She was very concerned with the rapport between Dr. Colp and the staff as a result of this experience.

SY: The following day I took care of Mrs. Abel again and typically she immediately began to complain about the previous night. I was greeted with a steady stream of complaints. I thought this must be the thing that really gets the nurses down because what this does is to make the nurses feel inadequate. I almost wanted to say, "Please don't do it this way, you make the nurses so angry."

SA: The nurses were now very angry. This is when Elaine kept saying to me, "I'm just living for my days off." And they all got very irritable, very sharp with each other, "I'm living for my days off to get away from all this."

SY: Anyway, breakfast came up again and again we went through the routine of being nauseated. I said, "Come on, let's try the cereal," or "If you don't like it, don't take it." So we talked about pleasant things and she ate, and I thought: "My God, she's just like a child." I'm standing there like Mama saying, "You eat your breakfast like a good little girl," and she would eat for me, and this would be continued for the rest of the month.

SA: Did you have any difficulty in getting out of the room?

SY: Yes. This was the second morning I was taking care of her, and I was going through the supreme test of one request right after another. Even though I kept telling her I was going to be with her all morning, she needed to use these tricks. Later she didn't have to do this, but I was really put through the paces that morning.

SA: Yes, I have notes reporting that Elaine said you always planned to leave at 12:00 but never left until 1:00.

SY: That's true.

SA: And then Elaine put an aide in her room for the rest of the afternoon.

SY: Anyway, after breakfast she wanted an orange peeled, so I peeled it for her, and she began to reminisce about happy Christmas times when she was a child and looked forward to eating. They used to decorate the Christmas tree with oranges and apples. Then she began to cry, saying that kids don't know what they're missing today, that it's nothing but tinsel, glitter and tinsel, that's all Christmas trees are. Then I said, "Does recalling happy times make you sad?" She didn't answer. She continued to weep for a while.

Then she said her back itched, and I would put some ointment on? I said sure, and found the ointment. She gave very elaborate instructions on how to squeeze this ointment tube: you held it this way and you pushed it this way. I was fascinated. That morning I was so wary that I had to play games with myself, saying, "Here's a new ritual." (Everytime I would go in I would kind of play games, anticipating the ritual she had dreamed up or probably had all along.) Then I started putting on the ointment and all of a sudden the construction equipment outside the hospital began banging away. She wanted me to close the windows. So, here I am, my hands all messy with this ointment, and I say, "Just a minute, I'll be through in a minute." She insists on closing the window. I laughed and said, "I'll be through in just a minute." She started to cry and insisted. It became a matter of wills between us. When she began crying and insisting, I was really finished. I was glad it was over because I don't think I could have tolerated this battle of wills. I closed the window. I saw that this must be the kind of thing that she does, this power struggle that drives nurses mad. You don't know how far you should go—where you put your foot down and whether you go on with the gag. I made a notation at this time of "Where does one set limits and how?" This is the thing I am struggling with.

SA: Mrs. Abel was trying to get me to put on that ointment during the same period. Because of her medication, I think, she had really begun to tingle and itch. Every so often she would bring up this ointment, and I had the feeling she was really asking me to put it on. I never did. I always got one of the nurses to do it. I was trying to stay out of the nursing role per se.

SY: The other thing that fascinated me about this ointment was that she would press the tube a certain way, and when she pressed it the ointment would be sucked back into this tube. She just seemed divided because it was retracted back again. "How important it must have been for her to be able to control" was what crossed my mind when she became so divided that when she squeezed it one way it would retract, and when she squeezed it another way it wouldn't.

Then when I gave her an enema that morning, it was another struggle. She was very constipated because of the heavy narcotics and also because she just wasn't moving around much. I thought I was being real smart, you know, I was going to clue her in and we'd plan this thing together. I gave her the enema. She sits on the commode, and I check back on her every few minutes but she's not doing much. About fifteen minutes after I had given it to her I find her sleeping. I woke her up and said, "You are going to have to expel this enema." So she points to the chair and said, "Sit down and talk to me." I was sort of startled. Thinking, "*Nobody* wants to have people observing them when they're expelling an enema," and it occurred to me then that really she is like a child. I stood by her again I was playing the Mama role, saying, "You be a good little girl and expel your enema." And she chatted with me and expelled the enema. It occurred to me that these must be the things that startled and irritated the nurses who'd have to play this kind of role with the patient.

AS: I'm wondering if you really asked the nurses whether these were the kinds of things they reacted to?

SY: No, because when I got the facts and began to find out nobody wanted to talk to me about the patient. They "wanted out."

SA: I noticed, too, that it was then Mrs. Abel began to sleep and couldn't remember when she had her medication. She started to ask the nurses to remind her to cross out the medication in her notebook. She came even to that point! The nurses felt she was no longer legitimating her pain: she was sleeping through it, and very definitely she was. She was so confused with the massive doses of narcotic that she couldn't even remember to cross things out in her book This put the nurses in even more . . . they couldn't tolerate the notebook in the first place and when Mrs. Abel started asking them to remind her to take care of the notebook, this was sort of last straw. They had really begun to question the amount of emotional pain and the amount of physical, organic pain. They believed she was emotionally overreacting. This kind of distinction is sort of intermingled around the middle of November until December 6, when they actually pull out.

*   *   *

This is a continuation of December 3. I was telling about Mrs. Abel expelling the enema. Mrs. Abel's bath was one of the most involved procedures I had ever seen. There were two basins, one to wash certain parts of the body with and the other to wash other parts. And one was to rinse with. I was fascinated by this fancy procedure. She went into a long explanation as to why the bath had to be this way. Before she started the bath, she lifted up her edematous arm and said, "I wonder how much it weighs." I said, "You wonder about it," and Mrs. Abel said she wanted to know how much her arm weighed so that she would know how much weight loss she actually had, because her weight in the morning was very deceiving since actually most of the weight was in the arm. She gave most of her bath to herself, and through all of this she carried on a steady stream of conversation, one topic leading into another. There wasn't a pause, I couldn't even say "uhuh," or ask for any clarification. I did ask for clarification by saying "you said earlier . . ." but she always maneuvered me, so I gave up. I found this constant talking extremely wearying. For one thing I'm not fond of garrulous people. There were times in the morning when I felt 'Gee . . .'"

But I realized that this was a means of controlling the nurse, keeping the nurse at the bedside. I asked the nursing staff if this went on all the time, and they said, "My God, yes. We go to the patient's room and you try to leave but she carries on a conversation and you say, 'I have something to do, I have another patient to take care of,' but she would say, 'Let me finish this story,' and this contact would last another ten, fifteen, or twenty minutes." They were complaining bitterly about this. Then the bathing: she had to wash her ears four times and all the bodys parts were meticulously washed. Again, this fascinated me because I thought this is what she does. These are the mechanisms she uses to keep the nurse at the bedside. I asked the staff if this was the usual procedure, and they said, "My God, yes, a nurse goes in there and she ties her up for two or three hours just giving a measly old bath."

About 11:00 time was running out, and I told her that I was leaving at 12:00. Suddenly she looked at the time and said, "The percodan, you forgot to give it to me." I had given it to her earlier and hadn't let her write it into the book. I told her that I had given it to her on time. Her answer was that she got so many pills that she was drowsy and lost track of time, while actually she was very alert and talking rapidly. After she said this I felt bad because I realized that what I was doing was humiliating the poor woman, and actually I was in a way denying that she really did have pain. There were two things that I was trying to find out: did she really have as much pain as she said and she had; and can she be distracted? After that I decided that there wasn't any sense in humiliating her and let her write in the book whenever I gave her the pill.

The dawdling continued at the bath, and by this time I was getting pretty irritated. I said, "I'm getting awfully irritated with this," and told her I was leaving at noon and that there were certain things that needed to be done. There was still the breast dressing that had to be changed. She looked at me innocently and said she didn't know what time it was. I thought, "How do you beat a situation like this?" I asked the staff if this kind of thing went on all the time. They answered, "Oh yes, you know, you get manipulated all over the place." I was thinking how sad for this poor women, she wants love and yet she does the very things that make people reject her.

Anyway, getting back to the kind of conversation that went on. She talked further about her poor relationship with her husband. She repeated over and over her high sense of beauty and regret about not pursuing art. Several times in the morning she talked of her desire to die and, at the same time, of her hopes about the new drugs that the doctor was trying.

SA: This is the same format she used with each new person who appeared on the scene. She did it with me, the chaplain, Shizu, the social worker—right down the line.

SY: She recounted all her physical illnesses, very minutely, and then she talked about her whiplash injury. She went on with great anger about being cheated out of a reasonable settlement. She felt that it was the whiplash which hastened the cancer process. It was the anxiety and the stress—these are the two words she used—which caused the dormant cancer to flare up. She had read in a woman's magazine that there is a relationship between stress and anxiety to the growth of cancer, because what it does is causes hormonal imbalance, I listened to her and thought, she has to have some explanation of why the cancer is progressing. Periodically she would cry about. . . . Then she went on to say that she believed things happen to a person for a reason. She dwelt on this for some time. She talked about her religious beliefs, about reincarnation, and again over and over that whatever happens to a person is for a reason. I almost got a feeling that what she was saying was that whatever happened to a person is like a punishment. That was the feeling I got.

SA: Yes.

SY: Then she said she would like to be reborn a human again because she had some pretty bad luck.

SA: She also said she didn't want to be reborn again if she had to go through *this* again: the disfigurement and pain.

SY: Then she talked about how she took care of her mother before she died, what a wonderful mother she was, how hard she worked to make her mother's last days more comfortable, and she said this over and over again. I wondered as I listened to her if she had had death wishes about her mother and if this was guilt provoking? She had reason to have those wishes because she was brought into this world luetic and deformed.

Then I asked about the social worker. She brushed it aside saying that so many people came to see her that she really didn't know what happened. Checking back with the social worker later, I discovered they'd had a rather extended discussion about the possibility of discharge.

Then in the course of the morning she offered me a lipstick that she had been using—she could cut the end off and I could use it. I told her I had plenty of lipsticks and didn't need it. Later she offered me a little book, the kind she keeps her narcotic records in. I told her, "I really don't have any use for it." At the end of the morning she said, "You've been so nice to me, won't you please take a dollar." I told her I appreciated her feelings but she really didn't have to bother. She started to cry. "I want to give you something but you won't take it." I asked if she was real upset about it. All of a sudden the tears stopped and she said, "Shizie, when are you coming back again?" I told her I was coming back next week and would be coming in two mornings a week. I guess I should have taken the gifts, yet I had a feeling that she didn't have to buy me. Also I didn't want to be controlled by her in this manner.

Then I reported off. I was interested in finding out if other people felt the way about Shirley arousing Mrs. Abel by questions about pain that Helen did—she had made the comment about Shirley— so I asked the head nurse. She felt that Mrs. Abel became more agitated when all these people who were doing studies on her came to talk to her. "I find the nurse who is doing the pain study annoying too." I asked her what she meant. "Mrs. Abel seems to be more agitated and has more pain after Shirley has seen her because there is more focusing on pain. She's *impossible* after this nurse talks to this patient."

AS: Who were all these other people doing the studies?

SY: Actually there was one other nurse doing a study. . . .

SA: Another student who was doing a study on interviewing and technique and using Mrs. Abel. One of the basic students.

SY: There was another graduate student doing a study on expectations of what this illness was going to do for the patient's later life. I asked, "What are you doing with Mrs. Abel?" She said, "Oh, I talked to her for a very short while and dropped her because I realized she wasn't a very good candidate." So actually there weren't that many people seeing the patient.

SA: At first they didn't know what I was doing, and the head nurse never talked to me nor was she ever around when I was on the floor, which was three-quarters of the time.

SY: Anyway, during this conversation two of the nurses came up. I caught Helen and got her involved. One other nurse and the vocational nurse came up, and I asked them questions. They all agreed that Mrs. Abel did have more pain after Shirley visited her.

SA: The word used then was that she was "preoccupied" with pain.

AS: We made a mistake in not explaining to the nurses that we did not talk about pain with Mrs. Abel.

SA: I did, but not with the head nurse because I never saw her. That was the new head nurse who came during the middle of the study. I told her briefly what I was doing and saw her only two or three times the entire time I was on the floor. She was either off or away from the floor and I rarely spoke to her.

When Shizu told me and I decided to pull out, I talked to Elaine about why I was pulling out. There seemed to be some concern that when I was talking to Mrs. Abel, I was focused on pain. I said, "You know, Elaine, I never said a word to her." I walk in and say good morning and she talks as she did the other day, for an hour on the weight of the magazine, due to the amount of advertising, or some other subject. Pain never came up. I purposely did not mention the word just to see whether Mrs. Abel would bring it up or not. Elaine said, "Yeah we know." It was then that the girls gave me the feeling that they didn't want me around. We still had a good relationship, and I pulled out to maintain it, in order that I could go back at intervals.

Actually, I talked to the nurses at intervals. I didn't stop talking with the nurses. But I pulled out from seeing Mrs. Abel with the excuse that Shizu had given me that maybe there were too many people involved.

SY: I ran into the chaplain on that morning, and his comment was, "Isn't she something, though? We exchanged information and it was pretty much the same information that the patient had rattled off to me during the morning. I was interested, however, in knowing that the patient had bared her bosom to the chaplain the first time they met, just as with me. Later I found out she did the same with the social worker.

AS: The patient was doing exactly the same thing with everybody although depersonalizing the whole process of contact with everybody. She was building up a common imagery that everybody could share—one which they could talk about in somewhat denigrating, horrified terms. In other words, whenever they piece together information they all discover that everyone has been told the same things or had the same experiences. They can't help but form a common imagery about her rather quickly. Do either of you have any impressions about this?

SA: I'm sure of it.

AS: The chaplain's indication to you, Shizu, sounds like you've gotten this impression too. And people greeting each other: "Oh, it's your turn this morning." You probably heard this all over the unit. Did you?

SA and SY: Yes.

SY: People would use the phrase, "You know what I mean."

At the end of the week I wrote this: "Mrs. Abel is indeed a disturbed and disturbing patient. This illness with all its fearful meaning exaggerates her past neurotic behaviors. It is obvious her behavior is regressed—dependency, with whining, and wanting constant attention. The nurse must play a mother surrogate role, but it is all consuming and sometimes very, very hard to take. The breast cancer is a further threat to her already badly damaged body image. Her illusion of sensitivity to beauty and artistic abilities are long standing defenses for the damaged image. Her elaborate record keeping is a method of controlling the environment. Pain is exaggerated in her case because of the threat of breast cancer on an already damaged body image. Pain seems to be symbolized in guilt, punishment, and aggression which intensifies pain. The rituals are very important to her, and I am up a tree, not knowing where one interferes with it and where one does not. I need help in trying to know what to do in relating to the patient and also in terms of managing the patient.

AS: Two questions: first, did you ever see anything approximating this kind of language in the chart?

SY: No.

AS: The other question, did they ever call in a psychiatrist?

Was there ever any talk about this? Did either of you bring that suggestion up?

SY: I raised it later.

SA: When Dr. Colp was telling me about not knowing what to do with her—before he made her a research patient—he said he had thought of a psych consult but had decided not to have one because of the length of time that she would live. He had decided a consult would have little therapeutic value. It wasn't worth it for her to undergo therapy, at this point, it would take too long.

SY: To continue: I was quite frustrated. I really felt that I needed some help. I needed expert psychiatric help. And I made arrangements to find out what Mrs. Abel's physician felt about it. The other notation I made was that Mrs. Abel had the right to all her "defenses," but unfortunately these defenses repelled the nurses. And that it was sad to see her dying unloved, distraught, and without peace. I wrote that I can't say that I was therapeutic to the patient, and I'm not sure I can be realistically. Anyway, then I felt I should talk to somebody. The instructor wasn't around so I made arrangements to talk to the social worker and the cancer research nurse the following day, because obviously I could not talk to the rest of the staff in objective terms. This was now December 3.

SA: June and I talked earlier about the extensive terminology that Shizu was using and also about the need for some ability and skill (in terms of psychiatric orientation) to be able really to take care of Mrs. Abel. June was frustrated, she left she didn't have this kind of skill. She's the only one that I picked up this kind of informatior from.

AS: Is she the only college trained nurse on that unit?

SY: No, Helen is, too. . . . I saw Mrs. White, the cancer research nurse on our faculty. We discussed Mrs. Abel, mostly my frustrations about the patient and trying to find out if it was possible to get me a psychiatric consultation. Mrs. White was encountering some difficulty. Also she was trying to get some of the psychiatric nurses placed on the unit. She felt that such things as improved in-service regular psychiatric consultation, and staff meetings were necessary on the unit.

Then I saw the social worker. She was happy to see me because when she had announced to the nursing staff that Mrs. Abel's stay might be extended, the nurses moaned and groaned saying they couldn't possibly put up with Mrs. Abel any longer. Incidentally, she was not the regularly assigned social worker. She is working on her master's degree and has a student role at the hospital. We exchanged information. She felt that she was running into difficulties in making discharge plans with Mrs. Abel's doctor because his plans were so indefinite. She was surprised when I said the doctor was thinking of continuing hormone therapy with this patient. She believed that Dr. Colp was telling the nursing staff one thing and another thing to the patient—telling Mrs. Abel that they were extending her stay while telling the staff he was making plans to have the patient discharged. The social worker said that there were two alternatives open to Mrs. Abel, both of which she rejected. To go home or go to a county hospital. When I asked her what I might do to help the situation, she said, "As much as Mrs. Abel hates to face reality, the reality is that she has to eventually face the fact that she must leave the hospital. So it would help if she can be brought to reality, if you get her to discuss this with you." I said that it was extremely difficult to get the patient to discuss this, as she was very adept at manipulating the conversation and was denying any thought of going home. She had been with the case a very short period, by the way.

AS: The patient never went home, so it would have been unrealtistic to tell her that she was going home—as things turned out. The social worker just assumed that reality was as she herself saw it.

SY: Yes, Mrs. Abel looked pretty good. Dr. Colp was now thinking in terms of the patient living for maybe six months. Then the social worker said there was a conference planned with the husband, the patient, and herself. I asked if I could be involved, and she said that would be fine. She had been having a difficult time trying to pin Mrs. Abel down as to when her husband was available or when he could be reached. It got the same impression.

SA: I have in my fieldnotes at that time, Shizu, that you had already begun to see Mrs. Abel as terminal. You remarked that you felt more and more agitated as the end came closer. This was December 4. You were still standing on the outside, looking in, and very amused about Mrs. Abel's various ritualistic patterns, and waiting to see what happened next.

This was when Elaine had talked about their being very choppy when they left Mrs. Abel's room. They began telling of their feelings about Shizu and about a situation which happened after Shizu left one night, although she stayed until about 1:00. Elaine has to put an aide in the room for twenty-five minutes with Mrs. Abel, giving pills, changing her dressing—the whole ritual. "I don't know how long they're going to keep her here. Breast tumor isn't the burning problem any longer, and the tumor board isn't learning anything from her." Dr. Colp was just keeping her in. This was the 4th of December. Two weeks later, she was really pushing to get this patient out and was telling the supervisor about it. Also, Elaine then almost had hatred for the patient, because she described another lady to me: "That lady was nothing. A year ago, she was a big problem and I used to go through a ritual with her where I'd bring her a cookie I had made the night before at home. I'd do anything to have that lady here instead of Mrs. Abel because she showed appreciation for the ritual and Mrs. Abel does not." So there was a great deal of feeling about Mrs. Abel.

SY: Their amusement began to appear around the middle of December. It was pretty high amusement. "Did you hear about the other particular thing that she did"—this sort of thing.

During team conference on December 5, I asked the nursing team if they had any suggestions about what I or they might do to relate better to the patient. This drew no suggestions. I got the feeling that they were up a tree. And I was up a tree. I gathered they were fed up and didn't want to discuss it. They would discuss it in terms of laughing derisively about it, and so forth, but not in terms of what actually could be done.

Again we went through this ritual about the patient being nauseated and not being able to keep anything down. So I stayed with her, and she talked and ate almost everything off the tray. I thought, "I'll involve her more and discuss what we're going to do this morning and see if this will make any difference, see if the dawdling would change." It didn't make one bit of difference. Mrs. Abel talked and talked and talked, pretty much about the kind of things she talked of before. I made no effort to ask for clarification, and she would repeat the same things over and over again. I checked back and asked the staff if this was the kind of thing she did. "Yeah, drives you nuts. The same old story morning after morning." But somehow this morning I felt differently about her talking: If she stops talking she will lose contact and so she has to keep it up. It wasn't nearly as irritating as the week before.

SA: Notice the flavor of this! Shizu began to interpret, digging up motivations for why Mrs. Abel did varying things. She also began to try varying tactics, then sat back to evaluate them to see if they would work—or what they would do to Mrs. Abel. Let her talk, try to follow her ritual on pills, and then evaluate. Shizu, you began to get a little frustrated about "what can I do for this woman; really, I haven't found anything that works."

SY: Periodically Mrs. Abel would complain about pain and weep about its uselessness. However, I did notice that she did not complain about it as much as the week before. Again, the medicines were given exactly on time, and I allowed her to record them. It occurred to me, what could the nurses have done earlier during the course of her care? If they had done something differently would her focus on pain be less? Yet I couldn't decide what the nurses could have done. Such things were running through my mind.

During the morning she said she was going to go home. I thought, "Aha, I'll pursue this"! "You're planning to go home?" She said, "Well, of course, eventually everybody plans to go home." I pursued this further, and she kept telling me how Dr. Colp was planning some new hormones which she hoped would help. She said Dr. Tree was planning some studies on her. When I asked when the doctor was going to start these, she said she didn't know. I pursued this further, and she said she didn't know when it was starting. She repeated how she hoped this would retard the process. I pushed it further, and she said she couldn't go home because her husband is so inadequate. I thought, "She can't pursue it, and I'm not going to fight this issue with her. I'm going to let the social worker handle this problem."

AS: Did it ever occur to you that this woman was really trapped, and when?

SY: Yes. About two weeks later I thought there was no sense in trying to bring this up. She couldn't see any way out. . . . The social worker came when I was upstairs and began to discuss plans to meet with her husband. After a lot of hedging Mrs. Abel was finally pinned down to a date when her husband could be reached. She began to cry and said, "I can't be worried about my husband. Maybe I'm acting like a big baby, and I'm lost in self-pity, but with my condition I'm entitled to self-pity." The social worker stated that the patient had the right to these feelings but that they had to come to some solution that all parties could agree to mutually. After the social worker left, the patient wept a lot for about fifteen minutes. I could not do anything for her except to let her cry. I reported off to the team leader who was merely interested in knowing when the next narcotic was due and not really about what went on with the patient. I asked what she had done in terms of trying to relate better to Mrs. Abel. She said, "Nothing works. Do whatever you like. You do whatever you think is right. I don't care what you do."

This was when I put down, "I feel very frustrated. I'm getting nowhere. I feel like I need psychiatric help." Then the chaplain came to the class seminar and a goodly portion of the discussion was spent on Mrs. Abel again. I don't think we came to any solution though. The gist of the seminar was mostly his role in helping the dying patients, and how the chaplain and nurses could work as a team in helping patients. Mrs. Abel was brought up as an example!

On December 6 Mrs. Abel was quite nauseated from all the drugs she was on, so promazine was given. Doctor Colp made the notation on her chart, "Possible discharge. Discussion with patient in a few weeks. The patient might become anxious." Mrs. Abel was getting more depressed, so the doctor gave her some drugs as a mood elevator.

SA: This was when Elaine really started wanting to get rid of Mrs. Abel. By this time Dr. Colp had started pulling off the floor—because Elaine was asking *me* for information. Elaine was the assistant head nurse who was really running the floor. She had got the information concerning Dr. Tree from me before. You see, they were waiting for Dr. Tree to come back and complete his studies. She knew that I had obtained the information before, so she asked me again if I knew anything about where Dr. Tree was. She didn't know he was away. By this time, I did because I had double checked. She thought Dr. Tree had been seeing the patient and that maybe there would be two more weeks of therapy and then two weeks to get her ready for discharge to County or somewhere. Then they would be getting rid of her. Elaine said Mrs. Abel had got them like puppets on a string. "She's really gotten to us and we just act like puppets and do whatever Mrs. Abel wants us to do. Dr. Colp doesn't want to discharge her. . . . I can't see throwing her out in the cold snow, but . . ." and her "but" just hung. She said Dr. Colp felt sorry for Mrs. Abel and is really vague when he talks about her. We can't pin him down to anything. I think it was that day that she wanted me to pin Dr. Colp and Dr. Tree down to find out exactly what was going on. The nursing staff was getting quite desperate to get her out and afraid she might stay forever. They said in the afternoon report that Mrs. Abel was just impossible to handle. Elaine told me she talked to the supervisor about it. In other words, the nurses had become desperate in about three or four days. The supervisor had told them that she would continue pushing Dr. Colp for the discharge; but that her hands were tied unless Dr. Colp did something about it. She would pressure him, but he had to write the order. . . . This was when the nurses indicated, too, that Mrs. Abel was feeling lousy at night that she was annoying the other patients.

AS: It's important to see here that they hadn't yet realized that Mrs. Abel was terminal; therefore there's no end to her stay on the floor—the research could go on forever. And they would all be in anguish if it went on forever.

SA: They were getting really desperate. One girl said, "Mrs. Abel is so self-centered," and they began to categorize her with this type of terminology. She does not want to leave here, and she said she won't get the expert care at the County Hospital that she was getting at this hospital. Mrs. Abel used this tactic to keep the nurses in the room.

SY: I remember Elaine saying, "She's *so* selfish" with great anger I think she *said* to the patient, "I think you're so selfish."

SA: In fact, the chaplain got around to telling Mrs. Abel, "Try, maybe you could set a better example for the other patients on how to accept suffering." This was the 1st of December, and he was trying to change . . .

SY: After a lot of chasing around, on December 9 I finally located Dr. Colp. I was interested in his plan of therapy. I also wanted to know if there was a possibility of psychiatric consultation. He had just seen the patient and had told her about eventual discharge. He expected the patient now to become quite agitated. He was waiting for Dr. Tree's return from vacation to discuss the possibilities of new pain studies, and therefore Mrs. Abel's discharge would be delayed for about a month. He mentioned again the problem of discharging Mrs. Abel because there were only two possibilities—home or to the County Hospital. He was very disturbed that the County Hospital wanted a lien on Mrs. Abel's house, and he didn't think this was fair. He had questioned Mrs. Abel at great length about the pain in her arm. He felt that it was actually a heaviness, not pain. He said the pain Mrs. Abel described was like a dullness and a heaviness experienced after novocain injection in dental work. There was no pain as such but one could feel the pulling and tugging. This was not pain. He assured the patient that no matter what drugs they gave her, they could not stop this feeling.

SA: This is the first time *this* point came up. Before he was reassuring her that they will take care of her pain. Now he's saying that they can't. That same day, he indicated to me a feeling of depression about county hospitals: she just wouldn't get as good care there because those places are always so depressing. He explained the lien a little further, saying that it will be used to pay the county hospital bill, and this wasn't fair to the husband. This was a persistent attitude of his—to take all the money that people have saved for a home to pay for an illness. He constantly mentioned this. He said he was definitely going to wait for Dr. Tree's return. Dr. Tree was the justification for keeping Mrs. Abel in the hospital. He emphasized this again: he's keeping her despite the nurses and that the budget is getting very low. He was actually turning other patients away, not admitting them, and just cutting corners with other patients except for Mrs. Abel.

AS: Let's go back just for a moment to the conversation he had with Mrs. Abel about the heaviness and tightness. Is this the first time we know of that he has told her there is nothing he can do about this? He's also telling her it's not really pain. Does she believe it?

SY: No, because the following day I questioned her at great length about what the pain was like, and she kept saying it's a heaviness and, "It's a real pain." She kept saying, "I really have pain," over and over again.

SA: I would say she probably did not believe the explanation because she used the same tactics to prove that she had pain. And Dr. Colp said, "Even if I had this tightness, I, *too,* might have expressed this as pain. She always expressed this as pain."

SY: Then I asked the doctor if the patient ever had psychiatric help and the possibility of getting psychiatric consultation. He sounded quite hostile as he said, "Do you think it's going to help her now?" I answered that I certainly didn't think it would help her in any long term way, but I did feel that the psychiatric consult might be able to help her in some way. Also, I said that the nursing staff needed it, and I, too, needed help in terms of relating to the patient. He didn't think it would help: "Maybe *you* take your problems home with you, but *I* don't because I forget her the minute I get off the station." I thought to myself, "The hell you do."

AS: Was he aware that the chaplain was trying to act like a quasi-psychiatrist to the patient?

SY: No, but he knew that the chaplain was seeing her.

My feeling was, "I bet you take Mrs. Abel's problems home with you because I remembered in last week's discussion when you mentioned that you had a problem similar to this in your family and there was nothing you could do about it." And I thought he must really find this a threat and wondered if he was running into problem with pain pills and all the related moral and ethical problems. So I asked again, "Then you're saying that you don't think psychiatric consultation would help?" He said no, that he was not psychiatrically oriented anyway. Then he went on to say that the patient had fecal impaction a few days before and wanted him called for digital removal, but fortunately he was not available. The nurses refused to do the digital removal. (I, myself, didn't know

96

what I would do under the circumstances if I were faced with this problem.) Then he looked down at the medication charting sheet and said, "Well, there are a few more free spaces available to order more drugs. She's getting enough pills now, but there are three more spaces." By this point I was getting pretty irritated with him. "You keep treating her and treating her, giving her a lot of false hope, and probably just relieving your own conscience." The doctor was getting irritated by me, too. He looked down at his watch and said he had to see another patient on another ward. At this point I wrote in my notes, "I wish I knew what to do; I'm stuck."

SA: I didn't talk to you until a couple of days afterward. When the three of us got together on December 9.

SY: On that day the doctor discontinued some of the other drugs he had been treating her with for cancer—ACTH and the tyroid—and started estrogens.

On December 10 I debated whether to continue taking care of Mrs. Abel as I didn't seem to be getting anywhere very fast. But I decided Mrs. Abel probably could tolerate some unirritated nursing care. I decided that I would have no plan of care but merely be with her and give her what little comfort I could give her. I told the team leader that I would take care of her total medications (where previously I had only been responsible for the narcotics). She very happily relinquished this task to me.

Mrs. Abel was very sleepy and quiet all morning. Her silence bothered me. I wondered if the discussion with Dr. Colp about eventual discharge made her quiet and if sleep was a way out of thinking about it. I asked several times during the morning if something was bothering her because she was so quiet. Each time she would say she was drowsy from the medications. Actually she had not been receiving more than the usual amount.

When I questioned her about the pain in the arm, she said again it was a dull, aching pain. It never went away and it was really very painful. I asked if the social worker had been to see her, and she stated that a meeting was set for the following day at 3:00. I asked if I might sit in on it. She wanted to know why, and I told her that I was interested in knowing what happened and how I might be able to help. There seemed to be no objection; there seemed to be no surprise or even pleasure that I was intrested. I asked if she had thought of any solutions and said if she wanted to talk about it we could, but she never bothered.

The medications I administered were taken without the usual fuss and crying. What I did do was tell Mrs. Abel about those that

97

she had to take immediately. The others I allowed her to take at her own speed, because she used to get about nine to ten tablets at one shot. I left the ward troubled with her silence because I didn't know what it meant. I didn't know whether it was good or bad. On December 11 I saw Mrs. White, a faculty member of the School of Nursing.

I had a discussion with Mrs. White, and I had told her about my needing psychiatric consultation. I felt a need for it. She said she had posed the subject of psychiatric consultation to the nursing staff, and the assistant head nurse to whom she talked rejected the suggestion completely, saying that the nursing staff could adequately solve their problems through the nursing team conference.

My regular instructor was out of town during the week and a half that I was first beginning to work with Mrs. Abel so Mrs. White and I discussed the feasibility of staffing conference at this time but wondered if the nursing staff's attitude was such that nothing could be accomplished.

I read my diary and thought, "Oh, my God." I had been discussing with Miss Flanagan the possibility of next semester's projected plans: maybe running some team conferences. But I wouldn't certainly use this patient as a jumping off point. It would be like jumping into a fire. . . . When I saw Miss Flanagan, she assured me that I was doing my best, that I had exhausted resources and not to feel badly. It was shortly after this that I ran into Shirley.

What did this conference with Mrs. White do for me? Nothing. I ran into Shirley and we discussed Mrs. Abel at great length. At the end, Shirley reassured me that I was doing my best and not to feel badly about it. Then I ran into you, and you said (in so many words), "You can't beat the system," that the system is creating the problems and *don't feel badly* about it! At the end of the day I thought, "By God, three people in the past hour have told me not to feel badly, that I have done my best. Well, I'm frustrated in the situation, but probably I'm the only one that doesn't feel *too* badly about it because I'm the only one that's actually going in and *doing* something with this patient."

SY: I put down in my notes, "As ineffectual as I am, it must be of some comfort to the patient to have somebody come in who is not as irritated. All I could do in this instance is to be with her without demanding any great changes in Mrs. Abel."

AS: Before we go on: Shirley, had you and I talked yet about what *you* would have done if you had been a nurse in the situation?

SA: That was about a week earlier and followed the session with June when *she* didn't know what to do. I said I didn't know either. You and I had discussed the idea of the team conference, saying it was too late for it to make any difference.

AS: Shirley was very disturbed and so I asked her, "What would you have done if you were in the situation as a staff nurse?" trying to show her that the way the hospital is constituted such situations are not one person's fault; and that while perhaps something could be done for such a patient, with the present setup of our hospitals, it is very difficult to do much.

SA: As a nurse I honestly didn't know what could be done for this patient at this point. I really didn't have any answers. We hadn't come up with anything. As I remember, we said that maybe at the end of the study we might have some possible suggestions. I felt that despite the advanced training I had gotten in the last couple of years, I didn't have any answer for the situation at all.

AS: We also reviewed the kind of teaching they'd given you in the advanced classes, agreeing that the suggested tactics would not work. Shizu, in fact, tried these various tactics and they didn't work. She got such tactics from that class-work.

SA: This discussion was related to June asking me about ideas for care and I said, "Look I went to Dr. Strauss. As far as nursing care, he doesn't know, and I honestly don't know." Of course, June thought I was getting supervision in terms of possibilities for care. So when Shizu came on the scene, we already knew that we didn't know what to do, and I was waiting around to watch what Shizu, an equal in training to myself, would do in the situation.

AS: After Shizu talked with me, Shirley and I talked a bit. Soon after I went out and saw Shirley and Mrs. White talking on a street corner. I took in the situation. Mrs. White was giving out with hopeless cliches and feeling quite helpless. I felt sorry for her. She was understandably some miles away from the reality of what was happening on the unit herself.

SA: I remember you laughing as you walked up to us, as you realized what we were talking about. I wanted to hear what Mrs. White had been telling you, Shizu. Because here was a woman who had had considerable experience and more education than either of us, and I was wondering — *you* were having problems and *I* didn't know what to do about it — what would *she* do about it. And here I was, getting the cliches, you know, the same old thing, and I thought, "We've been through this." It was also on the same day that Dr. Strauss and I talked about Mrs. Abel and then Shizu came up to talk about Mrs. Abel. And here we were now, standing on a street corner talking about Mrs. Abel, some twelve stories away from where all the action was taking place. It had gotten to that proportion!

AS: I remember also how helpless Mrs. White was feeling about it. Still she was so absorbed with it she had to talk about it.

SA: This was the same day that you and I discussed these possibilities: *Would the nurses finally come to realize that Mrs. Abel was now terminal,* and would she stay in the hospital until the end or would Dr. Tree come back to finish his research and then get rid of her? *Later on that day I found that they realized they were never going to get rid of her.* We had predicted that day she would stay. We *knew* it.

SY: I wasn't ready to buy that yet. Partly because I had been talking to the social worker who had been working on plans, although Dr. Colp was saying, "We're running out of funds," and so on.

I went on the unit to meet with the social worker and the husband. While we waited on the ward I talked to the patient who wept about the discomfort of her arm at great length. She said it was a dull, aching pain. Then she was silent for quite a long time and kept looking at her arm. I said, "It must be very difficult for you." She cried and said, "I pray and I pray, but it doesn't seem to help." I said, "The praying doesn't help you," and she said, "It helps sometimes but most of the time it doesn't." Then as if talking to herself, "I wonder what happens to the soul, it must look for something and not find it, just as we seek something in life and not find it." I answered "yes" and kept nodding my head and encouraging her to talk, but she would not talk any more. Then I asked if she had been able to talk over these matters with the chaplain. She had been and liked the chaplain a great deal: "He's very nice, but I think I can preach as well as he can." So I said, "Do you feel you could preach as well as he can?" She answered that she could and went on again about her religious beliefs and reincarnation.

SA: This is the period, the latter half of November and the first half of December, in which she spends a great deal of time thinking about the philosophical aspects of life. We had about an hour discussion on the philosophical aspect—reincarnation and what the Essenes were, and so forth.

AS: Do you know of other nurses who got involved in this way?

SA: I doubt if any did; they knew about the reincarnation, but I suspect they did the same thing as Shizu because they were never able to give me any details about it except that she talking about

100

reincarnation. They didn't appreciate her philosophical point of view.

SY: Then there was a change of plan: the social worker decided that they would not meet with the patient, only with her husband. I went down to the office where Mr. Abel was agitated and wringing his hands. He said he just could not have Mrs. Abel at home because he was upset and had had a nervous breakdown before. If it were not for tranquilizers he would fall apart. He kept saying over and over and over that Mrs. Abel upset him, he didn't know what he was doing.

AS: I think we might note that by now the patient had been relatively abandoned by everybody except Shizu and the doctor. The doctor was the person who somehow kept the whole situation going, and Shizu was making forays into Mrs. Abel's room. I assume the chaplain also was not giving up yet. The social worker . . .

SY: The social worker was beginning to see her more frequently.

AS: Yes, she was beginning to do something. The husband had given up. The nurses had pretty much given up, probably the interns also.

SA: The chaplain hadn't given up. He was frustrated and not able to acknowledge that maybe he couldn't stand the situation, but he was not making excuses for not going into her room. He said there was always someone there; that other patients needed him who were terminally critical also. He began to spend more time with other patients and was comparing them with Mrs. Abel. He was also complaining (December 13) about the inability of the girls on the floor to relate to Mrs. Abel. He said they are having difficulty because they identify with her; that they too could have cancer; they too could have this kind of pain, and so forth, and therefore they have become hardened and hostile. "It's a crying shame, they just can't stand her making demads on them. I haven't had time to spend with her, there are so many terminally ill on the 14th Floor making demands on my time."

SY: The social worker stated that there were three possible discharge avenues open. One was to discharge the patient home— which the patient rejected, although she said that Dr. Colp kept pressing about sending her home with a vocational nurse.

SA: It would have to be somebody, he said, that would be willing to work around the clock, because medications had to be given around the clock. He didn't see this as feasible unless it were a full-time, paid nurse and this wouldn't be possible financially.

101

SY: Yes, and that was impossible.

SA: Yes, because she had to have the narcotics. He was really on a hot spot. He never did get off of it. Somebody kept the pressure on him right up to the end.

SY: The second avenue open was the County Hospital—which was rejected. The third avenue was the nursing home, which he felt was a pretty good possibility at this point. Contra Costa County apparently was willing to take patients in her condition because their nursing homes are not full to the same degree as nursing homes are in San Francisco. Anyway, she made arrangements for the husband to meet the doctor by calling the head nurse to page Dr. Colp when Mr. Abel arrived on the station. Checking back later I found out Dr. Colp was not available and did not meet with the husband. The social worker kept reiterating to Mr. Abel that they could not make any definite plans until they really knew what Dr. Colp's feelings were, in terms of what kinds of facilities Mrs. Abel really needed. Then the social worker instructed the husband to call the Welfare Department in Contra Costa County for application.

SA: Doesn't this strike you . . . although Colp knew right along what kinds of care were necessary, why was it taking two or three weeks to get all this straightened out between him and the social worker?

SY: Well she kept saying she didn't know which end was up.

AS: I think he was playing a game with her, as well as with the husband, because he couldn't really make up his mind what to do. He was twisting and turning, not being able to make a real decision. He couldn't tell her this, yet all along he probably knew that he would keep her just as long as possible. There is no way of knowing whether my guess is accurate—he wouldn't know himself at this point. At any rate, it is not merely a case of mis-communication.

SY: The social worker was going through a state of confusion of not knowing what were the nursing needs of the patient because this would determine where she would go from the hospital.

AS: And she doesn't know this particular doctor. She is relatively a novice as a social worker. If she had had a longer period of working with him, or had been an older woman, maybe she would have handled him differently.

SA: He must have been confused, too, because you would talk to him one time and he just couldn't see himself sending her to the County or a nursing home, and then later he would be making arrangements again to have her go.

SY: The social worker said that both the doctor and the patient had some mistaken ideas about the lien business. She was looking into this matter and really it wasn't as horrible as both had been led to believe.

AS: Did she ever get it straightened out?

SA: Yes, but it was difficult to straighten out with Dr. Colp because at the time he couldn't stand to talk back to you, Shizu, he had already left you once. I couldn't catch him anyplace. He was in a real dither. We all had trouble getting him. He pulled off, he was no longer coming to the floor, I couldn't get hold of him. You couldn't get him.

SY: On December 12 when I went on the wards the assistant head nurse told me that Dr. Colp had definitely made arrangements to keep the patient for several weeks more, awaiting a pain study. She said, "I could have cried when I found that out. You know Dr. Tree isn't coming back for several weeks and so the pain study will be delayed, and we will have to tolerate her that much longer."

SA: Elaine was just beside herself and said, "This will ruin my Christmas vacation if she is going to stay with us. We can't get rid of her." This was about the 16th.

SY: I asked if there was any change in Mrs. Abel, she was so quiet the last time I saw her. The answer the nurse gave was that she hadn't changed a bit and was getting more and more demanding and more and more unreasonable. On that same day, Dr. Colp wrote on the patient's chart, "Patient must call for help when the patient is up in the chair or walking."

SA: Elaine told me there were specific orders written for Mrs. Abel to receive the medication and to be supervised in her reception of medication, because they got concerned about this lawsuit. The doctor was worried about either the medication or that if she got out of bed and fell they would be sued. He wrote an order saying she had to be supervised and the nurses had to be in the room. This is why he was keeping them in the room.

SY: Then I asked the assistant head nurse how she would feel about a psychiatric consultation, wondering if it would help (and I used the word purposely) in handling Mrs. Abel. She doubted that anything would help at this point. I found Mrs. Abel talking to a visitor of another patient whom she had apparently just met. Mrs. Abel was trying to talk the visitor into exchanging manicures. The visitor looked very embarrassed and obviously didn't want to do it. I laughed and said, "It looks to me like you are getting the short end of the stick." The visitor laughed and seemed relieved that she could get out from under. I checked later and found out that Mrs. Abel got this visitor to manicure her nails. I laughed about it when I stopped at the desk and I told Elizabeth about it. Elizabeth said, "She makes me so mad, she manipulates everybody." She then went on to say how Mrs. Abel wanted this particular kind of nail polish so they ordered it. They went through all this rigmarole ordering this nail polish and then Mrs. Abel suddenly decided she didn't want it, she wanted to get it changed to another color. "She makes me so mad, she manipulates everybody." All I could do was just laugh. What else could you do? Anyway I told Mrs. Abel I would be back after the holidays to take care of her. She was *very* specific about when I was coming back and so on.

SA: It was on the 16th that you and I and the chaplain had a three way conference in the hallway. Remember?

SY: Oh, yes, and Dr. Colp came into the picture.

SA: Dr. Colp had been down to see the patient, and the three of us had gotten together. (By this time the nurses couldn't tolerate the sight of me. I had told Elaine that Mrs. Abel was definitely going to remain in the hopital and she said, "This is going to ruin my vacation." She said that day, "She is just *never* going to get out of here." That was the answer to our question about when they would begin to realize she wasn't going to leave. From that point on, the nurses couldn't tolerate the sight of me.) I went up on the floor that day, the 13th. I left Elaine because she didn't want to talk to me and I thought, "I'm not going to antagonize her, I will go find somebody else. The chaplain came on the floor. He said he had been spending lots of time with Mrs. Abel. On the 16th, he and I again got together, and Shizu. All three of us stood in the hallway and everybody just passed us as though we were just so much furniture on the floor. Dr. Colp almost did also, but I hung out an arm and snagged him as he went by. He changed the subject almost immediately. He started telling me about the research that he was involved in, something or other to do with his kidney research, and he said only about two words about Mrs. Abel. That was all I could get out of him, he completely changed the subject, just literally. In the meantime, Shizu and the chaplain stood there talking about Mrs. Abel. They were both deeply confused.

SY: I think we were talking in terms of her becoming more and more agitated and nothing or anybody being able to help her; and that she was avoided more and more by the staff, so getting more and more agitated. And actually that Mrs. Abel was a "bad, bad girl" but bad, bad girl attention is better than no attention at all.

The mood of the conversation was general helplessness. I just needed someone to talk to because nobody else would listen to me.

SA: I went up on the 18th because I was going to be leaving town (Shizu had already left). I wanted to get the latest information. I knew that I couldn't press the girls because they couldn't tolerate me. I had figured this out already. But I was trying to keep some form of relationship with this floor so that I could get some information in addition to that of Shizu. So I fixed up a box of Christmas cookies as a Christmas gift because, knowing nurses, this is one way that you show appreciation to a group of nurses. So I had taken a whole box of homemade cookies and decorated the box and taken it in. They had just been putting up the tree on that floor. (At this hospital they start celebrating Christmas about six or seven days before. They do that with parties and with cookies. Even research workers get swept into the parties on occasion.) I had been swept earlier into a going away party for Mrs. Firestone, but now they couldn't even think of that as a possibility, I can assure you! So I gave the box of cookies to them, and a couple of the girls commented "thank you" and left. You know, they looked at the note on the Christmas card and put the box under the tree—and literally just left. I was fascinated. They *just could not* tolerate being around me at all. They simply left. Well, this left me with the secretary who said that Mrs. Abel is "snowed" all the time. She was still crying. The secretary said, "She could stay here for a year, I guess." The girls asked Dr. Colp when Mrs. Abel would go. He told them she would be there as long as she was of use—meaning research—and she could stay as long as a year. The secretary said, "I guess she will be here until she dies." This was the first one who really said what you and I had already. . . . My reaction was sort of, "Ah ha, it is here," what we had anticipated. There were a few other people floating around, the doctors and people there at the station so I changed the subject and chit chatted in order to maintain our relationship. That's the last fieldnote I have until the 3rd of January.

THEORETICAL COMMENTARY: THE PAIN

The last lines mark the approximate end of a phase of a lingering trajectory during which Mrs. Abel's claims to pain were at the center of everyone's attention. That phase has now ended. Somewhat earlier the physician had decided she was dying, so had the chaplain, and now the nursing personnel have reached the same conclusion. Although Mrs. Abel will continue to have and claim great pain, the staff's preoccupation with pain will now merge with another concern: how to give her the comfort care that is offered to all dying patients.

We turn now to a theoretical commentary on the earlier "pain" phase of Mrs. Abel's trajectory. The commentary consists of an analysis of the events—and of the general story of Mrs. Abel's deteriorating relationships with the staff—during this phase. Our analysis is directed mainly by a theory of pain, whose origin was discussed in our introductory chapters.

Earlier we noted that when patients are recognized as dying, the staff organizes its activities in terms of the perceived dying trajectory. Similarly, when a patient enters a hospital ward, the staff members quickly begin to form estimations of how much pain a patient has, whether it will increase or decrease, and at what rate. In short, they have pain "expectations"—and perceive the patient as having a pain trajectory. Patients may also have such expectations. Leaving aside for the moment how these expectations are formed, let us note first that the nursing personnel who attended Mrs. Abel conceived of their ward as a place where patients usually die without much pain Furthermore, patients with Mrs. Abel's kind of cancer—even when they are dying—tend to have relatively little pain. Consequently, the nurses and aides neither anticipated that Mrs. Abel would offer a great problem in pain management nor were ready to believe that she had as much pain as she claimed initially. The doctor gave her a little more credit than they, but also expected a relatively easy pain trajectory. The experiences of all the staff, especially the nursing personnel, with previous cancer patients played a major role in their evaluations of how much pain Mrs. Abel really had— no matter what she claimed— during the first months. To understand fully, however, why they were successfuly able to reject her claims it is necessary to analyze how pain is discerned and what a patient may have to do before his claims to pain will be believed.

Only the person who is experiencing ("feeling") pain can directly perceive it. Others must either rely on his report, trusting him, or use his gestures as indicators of pain. When the onlookers expect pain, then crying, groaning, grimacing, wincing, perspiring, or the clenching of teeth may easily convince them. If they do not expect him to have pain, then he must make his pain plausible. In effect, he must legitimate his pain. Under ordinary household circumstances, someone can remark that he has a headache and get others to believe him, but hospitalized patients are known to be unduly afraid of pain and quick to claim more than they have.

When Mrs. Abel began her attempts to convince the staff that

106

she really did have considerable pain—crying and "complaining"—she only managed to persuade them that she had little or at least much less than she pretended. The more she attempted to legitimate her pain during these first months, the more she gave the impression of being "overdemanding," of not being honest about her assertions. After her readmission, when she was insisting on even greater pain, the nurses discounted this because she would sleep right through the night or would forget her so-called pain when she became engrossed in conversation.

In Mrs. Abel's case, the physician and the nurses assessed the amount of her pain somewhat differently, and this discrepancy began to lead to certain difficulties. We need to be clear on the complex division of labor which is involved in this multiple assessment. First of all, the physician is the legitimate person to assess pain—even if he is not certain and chooses to accept the assessment of the patient. Only he can legitimately decide on the proper means for relieving the pain. Rarely does he carry out the relieving activity himself but delegates it to someone else: in the hospital he delegates the task to the nursing personnel. When he orders drugs, then the nurses can have little discretionary power, unless that is delegated to them as when they may reduce or increase dosage by agreement or by order. Because the nursing personnel spend much more time with the patient, they are, or think they are, in a better position to reassess the patient's pain. Their reassessments are much affected by the patient's reactions while they are administering drugs, as well as by his reactions while they are merely working around him. If patients are too stoic or seem unrealistically "complaining," then the nurses can be misled.

Mrs. Abel, like many patients, adopted certain tactics designed to insure that her own assessment of pain got proper relief. Her tactics worked to some extent, but also irritated and angered the nurses. When her drugs were due, or even earlier, she got on the buzzer. She was preventing any possible increase of pain, or appearance of pain perhaps, that would arise because of a gap between drug administrations. She kept an account of the dosage in her book as they were given, presumably to insure that she got the proper amounts and at the correct times. She queried the nurses about what drugs she was getting. She attempted to prevent man-made pain, warning nurses when they injected her or complaining when they hurt her. The staff saw her as playing one person and shift against another. She also stockpiled her drugs against the day when she might need them desperately.

The personnel used standard counter-tactics, routine modes of dealing with patients like Mrs. Abel. They discounted her complaints, turned a deaf ear to criticisms, gave her drugs at longer intervals than she imagined the physician had ordered, and spelled each other in the onerous task of ministering to her needs and demands. But even in her first weeks on the ward these tactics did not work too effectively. One reason was that Mrs. Abel was doggedly persistent in her complaining and in reminding them about her drugs. Another reason was that she complained to her physician who in turn carried some of the message to them, to their understandable anger. Their anger was fed by their belief that he was putting them "in a bind"—telling the patient one thing (he would control her pain) and telling them another (keep her comfortable but don't wake her up for drugs).

For the understandings about pain control which grow up between physician and patient are crucial in their impact on ward events. Certainly they were in Mrs. Abel's case. In effect, Dr. Colp had promised her at first to keep the pain under control, believing he could. So his patient began with the expectation, trusting him. When he sent her home, neither she nor her husband could properly handle the medications, in order to control the pain, therefore he readmitted her to the hospital. The physician even allowed her some responsibility in her own control of pain, permitting her to schedule medications to some extent. However, he ran into a problem with her relatively early—the same one that he encountered with the nurses—because he tried to negotiate with her about sleeping through the night ("We can't wake you up to give you medication."), but she insisted that she needed the medication. Since, in fact, she did sleep through the night and later right through the scheduled administration, while yet demanding medications and complaining about not getting them, the nurses' anger toward her and the physician increased. The physician then is also in a bind: he is trying to keep pace, through increasing dosages of drugs, with the patient's genuinely increasing pain, but is well aware of the mounting strain between the nurses and himself. Meanwhile, as early as November 16, he is balancing two trajectories: a dying trajectory and a pain trajectory. He is estimating roughly that Mrs. Abel will live six months, with little chance that she might be saved, and yet he is aware that her pain may outpace his efforts at control—or if not actually outpace then at least Mrs. Abel would keep up her demands on the nurses.

Crucial in his calculations also was the absence of responsible kin. Had there been someone at home who could have administered the drugs, the physician would have discharged her. If she were sufficiently wealthy, private duty nurses could have been hired. Since neither condition was fulfilled, the physician had only the option of sending his patient to the county hospital as a welfare patient.

At this point his personal feelings entered the story: because of certain events in his own past, he could not stomach the idea of sending Mrs. Abel to the county hospital. This is only the first of several times that his experiential career will crosscut the hospital career of his patient. All nursing personnel except one, however, have no such experiential career, so they begin what later becomes a virtual campaign, pressuring their nursing supervisor to rid the ward of Mrs. Abel. By now the patient had become what the researchers termed "the patient of the day." She was the staff's main preoccupation. The patient's claims to pain now flooded the staff much as the pain itself flooded Mrs. Abel.

In any event, the staff's efforts to get Mrs. Abel discharged failed because of Dr. Colp's tactic of making Mrs. Abel into a research patient. Thus her pain—as Dr. Colp perceived it—first got Mrs. Abel readmitted to the ward and then kept her there as a special patient. And again his promises to a trusting Mrs. Abel are important: he assured her she would be kept just as comfortable on research drugs as on the drugs she had been receiving.

Since pain as a general phenomenon not only has such properties as intensity, direction and rate, but also varies in when it "appears," it is important that Mrs. Abel claimed her pain was quite continuous. If not continuous, it was at least intermittently frequent—that is, every two or three hours, and generally just before her next drugs were due. Such continuity in pain symptoms and complaints about pain is hard on the nursing staff, even when complaints are uttered in low key and pain is minor. Since Mrs. Abel claimed intense and worsening pain and complained loudly for all to hear, the nursing staff found her an increasingly difficult cross to bear.

They reacted not only by spending less and less time within beckoning distance of the patient but by disengaging each other from her room when stuck there. They carefully arranged staff rotation, so that nobody would have to spend much time with her. They invented the tactic of persuading her to a window which looked out on the city, hoping that her attention would be distracted both from them and her pain. They also reacted by spending more time with a highly valued terminal patient than normally they would.

Then we began to see the appearance of an important phenomenon, which we shall term "the balancing of priorities." Thus a physician frequency will decide to withhold temporarily pain relief because medication might obscure certain diagnostic symptoms. Or he will balance the giving of opiates against the probability that their administration will hasten death. Or he will give a milder rather than a stronger pain reliever because the latter will make the patient too groggy or will decrease the respiration rate. During the course of a patient's decline, the physician will balance and rebalance pain relief against other priorities—and so will the patient, the nurses, and the family. In Mrs. Abel's case, we see her relatively early balancing her increasing pain against her life. "The few moments I'm free of pain aren't worth living for." Soon she is balancing being groggy or awake against pain, deciding in favor of a slight reduction in sedatives. It is worth emphasizing that such balancing goes hand in hand with negotiation. At the moment, Mrs. Abel is negotiating with her physician to cut down her medications; earlier he had attempted to negotiate a reduction of her narcotics, but she had refused him. Later they will negotiate about further balancing.

Around November 17, there appeared another important phenomenon: the nurses gave way on their management of Mrs. Abel's pain relief, ceding over to her a considerable measure of control. ("We've sort of given up, we give her anything she wants.") By now, she was regularly and deliberately ringing her buzzer for medications at least ten to fifteen minutes ahead of the time they were due. The visible battle over who should control pain relief had been at least partly won by the patient—even though the nursing staff continued to discount the amount of pain. (Her positive response to the research doctor's placebo only furthered their disbelief.) The nurses' lessened control stepped up the process whereby Mrs. Abel became further insulated (or "isolated"), since the nurses spent less time with her—even time devoted to attempting to control her pain relief and her general behavior. Nevertheless the conversation among them turned frequently on Mrs. Abel: she was still a source of frustration and anger—which occasionally spilled over to color their reactions to each other and of course toward Dr. Colp. It also affected their relations with the nurse researcher, whom they began to reject because she was associated with getting Mrs. Abel to focus more on pain. That rejection continues for many weeks.

Although the nurses had partly yielded control of pain relief, by no means had they given up their attempts to control Mrs. Abel's inappropriate behavior. In anger, one nurse told the patient to stop crying. "Look, crying just doesn't help you, so stop it." Indeed, coming down sternly on her became a staff tactic during this period. Nevertheless, Mrs. Abel was pretty much getting her way with the scheduling of the medications, despite the frequent discussion among the staff about "setting limits." She was still attempting to keep the nurses at her bedside for the many minutes it took her to down her medications. (This had the consequence that the nurses sometimes left before the medications were taken, leaving her an opportunity for the stockpiling of drugs, an opportunity she possibly used.) In fact, Mrs. Abel continued to keep personnel in her room, if possible, by using stalling tactics such as dallying over her bath or making various requests. During this period, then, the contest over "presence" in the room continues and even increases, although the contest over management of pain relief actually had lessened. Thus Mrs. Abel's success at inducing personnel to attend her, plus the physician's instructions that because she was on massive doses of drugs somebody now had constantly to be in her room, meant she virtually had a private nurse. Whoever was in attendance was also engaged in a contest to reduce the number of her requests, which tended to come one after the other. In this contest the nurses were at a further disadvantage, for after the physician had given his instructions, they could not easily escape the room as before. Meanwhile Dr. Colp was increasing the bind they were in because he was, unbeknownst to anyone (except the researcher), postponing any further increase of Mrs. Abel's drugs, balancing the potential decrease of her pain against more important priorities. Nevertheless, he had given up thinking there was anything more he could do for his patient other than to keep her relatively comfortable. He will discharge her, he believes, after Dr. Mott has finished his drug research with her.

About this time, November 25, the student nurse elected to care for Mrs. Abel, and in effect becomes a private duty nurse, giving occasional care to her. Unlike the staff nurses, the student perceived Mrs. Abel as a terminal patient—time of death uncertain and perhaps some months off. She had also a different ideology of pain. Pain was meaningful to a patient, and so a nurse should listen closely to a patient's complaints and comments. Mrs. Abel's tactics, as they focused around pain, presumably were associated with her anxieties and other psychological reactions, not merely with any need to dominate the staff. Listening and spending much time with Mrs. Abel, the student nurse heard the same details as the nursing staff did, but interpreted the pain as having to do with Mrs. Abel's changing body images. Her reading of pain was quite different from the staff's. She was not concerned with how much pain Mrs. Abel actually had or how much pain she could tolerate. She would even have been willing to admit that Mrs. Abel might have had little pain and yet assign it significance. The staff nurses, of course, perceived Mrs. Abel as having relatively little pain and thought it insignificant. On the other hand, the nursing care given by the student was much the same as the staff's, and Mrs. Abel's management of her was much like her management of the staff. Hence, she too found herself engaged in contests with her patient. Yet in describing Mrs. Abel's tactics, the student uses a more sophisticated—and ideological—language deriving from her training in psychiatric nursing. And since she saw her patient as dying, she had already moved ahead of the staff in defining her own actions as 'terminal care.'

By the time the student nurse had appeared on the ward, a collective story about Mrs. Abel had, of course, fully emerged. Details were continually added to the story, but its central theme remained constant: an immensely demanding patient, whose increasing pain was never fully legitimated. The student was heir to this story. She attempted to reinterpret its details; nevertheless from the beginning she too is caught up in its central theme. Her reinterpretaton of Mrs. Abel's acts and comments is more psychiatric, but her tactics do not work much better with Mrs. Abel than those used by the staff. Before long she also found that "nothing works." Both she and the staff were, in her words, "up a tree."

By now the staff was getting desperate because they envisioned that Mrs. Abel might be around forever, and yet could not get Dr. Colp to discharge her. They do not yet recognize that this frustrating patient is dying. They do not understand that the physician has disappeared from the ward mainly because he has nothing more to offer his patient.

By now Dr. Colp had gotten himself into financial straits because Mrs. Abel's prolonged stay was eating up his research budget. He was having to turn away potential research patients. To Mrs. Abel he also admitted that no matter what medications he gave, he could not stop the pain in her arm. He made a slight attempt to convince her that it was not really pain she was feeling, but of course was not successful. Shortly afterwards the student nurse accused him of merely dosing her and offering false hope—"and probably just relieving your own conscience." Their tempers were getting ragged because nothing seemed to work with this patient.

It is important to understand that the patient did not yet fully understand she was dying—or at least had not abandoned hope—and was still focused on her pain; whereas her physician and student nurse had moved to the next phase of concern with controlling pain in the context of dying. So had the chaplain, who though he now despaired of helping her psychologically or spiritually had not really abandoned her, anymore than had the physician and the student nurse. The nurses, however, could not yet feel the contradictory tugs of compassion and despair because they did not yet define her as "now dying." They do not yet perceive the pain as an indicator of death as an outcome. Since the social worker does not know Mrs. Abel was dying either, and does not understand Dr. Colp's attitude toward the County Hospital, she is confused and frustrated by his seeming vacillation about the discharge of his patient. Also, the chaplain and the student nurse were avoided by the nurses when each asked about Mrs. Abel, and both were much concerned about the nurses' avoidance of an increasingly agitated Mrs. Abel.

All these events were the consequence of a closed awareness context: some people did not know that others believed Mrs. Abel was dying, and the latter people intentionally choose not to reveal that their actions were based on those beliefs. The stage is now set for closed awareness to move into open awareness, when the nursing personnel will understand that Dr. Colp believes Mrs. Abel is dying. And so will Mrs. Abel. The closing scenes in Mrs. Abel's drama flow from a combination of open awareness and the staff's definition that the patient has reached the "nothing more to do" phase of her dying. Then there are new bases for disruption of the ward's work and sentimental orders—and of course for further deterioration of the relationship between Mrs. Abel and the staff.

A final word about the analytic commentary given in the above pages. Without a theory of pain, this commentary would have been much less pointed or specific, at least in the directions guided by the theory.

CHAPTER IV

THE LAST DAYS

This chapter covers the remainder of the lingering trajectory, that is the period of Mrs. Abel's stay at the hospital until her actual death there. The staff now understands that Mrs. Abel is dying, and so their preoccupation with her claims to great pain yield now to their concern over how to give her comfort care. But their mutual relationships continue to deterioriate, partly because of the cumulative preceding events, but also partly because this patient's dying trajectory is one of the most difficult types of trajectory for staffs to manage and endure.

STORY: THE LAST DAYS

AS: It was roughly from December 18 to January 3 that neither Shirley nor Shizu covered the case, except that Shizu saw Mrs. Abel on the 29th.

SY: I was up there observing for a Sociology class, and I dropped in to see Mrs. Abel. Mrs. Abel complained bitterly about the nursing staff, "You know, I try to be good by not making any

114

demands," but there were certain things she couldn't do for herself any more, and she hated to be in this compromising position. She cried for quite a period and then she said she didn't mean to be so demanding and wondered why she made everybody so angry with her. I said, "Well, what do you think might be involved?" She couldn't answer that. Then she said her hair was very dirty and needed to be washed. I told her that I would be by after the first of the year and would give her a shampoo. Again she pressed me for a specific date. I thought, "Well this hair is the only thing she has left, besides the nice fingernails," so I decided if this was going to comfort her I would do this.

Reading over the patient's chart I saw that the doctor noted that larger and larger doses of morphine had been required. The patient was on 300 milligrams of phenobarbital and this was raised to 64 milligrams of phenobarbital because she was getting more and more agitated. At the same time, she was getting more and more lethargic, so again they had to reduce it. During the Christmas week she had the morphine increased to 24 milligrams—and they were running into trouble because her respirations were becoming depressed. And there were periods when they had to withhold the morphine and the patient became very, very agitated. The patient's behavior had not changed. The nurse's notes said, "Upset about not receiving narcotics, crying, 'I wish I were dead, I can't stand it any more. I wish I could be put to sleep. All the medications just make me groggy but they don't stop the pain.'" One night she said to the night nurse while she was still groggy and asleep with the medication, "I see you have an elephant's hide, too." I stopped the staff to ask what had happened. They threw up their arms and said she was as bad as ever. I couldn't get any conversation out of them.

On the 3rd of January, when I came back after vacation, I went on the floor again talked to the secretary because I hadn't seen Shizu and I didn't know what she knew. The secretary said that everything had been relatively status quo. There had been very little change, very little difference in Mrs. Abel's behavior. "Oh, she may be a little worse." I also saw the chaplain. This is when he told her she ought to set an example for other patients, and Mrs. Abel's response to him was, "how much can I take?" His response had been, "I don't know, only God knows." Because he didn't know what this pain was, he didn't know what she could tolerate, and he didn't really know how to answer the question, this was his alternative answer.

He told me he really hadn't known what to say. "All I could think of to say at that point was I don't know and only God knows what you can take." And he said to me, "There really isn't any way

115

you can measure pain by using a yardstick." He also sort of apologized to me. "I have been neglecting her because there is always too many people there." This, I think, was in reference to my last discussion with him prior to Christmas when he told me he had been spending more time on the 14th Floor because (part of the reason) there had always been people in her room. I had pushed him: could it possibly be because he couldn't stand to go in and see Mrs. Abel? He didn't think so. Two weeks later he is analyzing that it could be a real possibility, or at least showing indication. . . .

AS: That he had thought about it? To him this is very important because this is part of his definition of his duty.

SA: That's right. Of course, by the time she dies it becomes even more important, because he literally does pull out and turn her over to a student.

AS: Yet this is the man who has held me spellbound for two hours giving me the details of how when everybody else more or less gave up on a patient he came crashing through, really doing a tremendous job of uniting the family, taking the patient over the threshold of death. This was one of his greatest professional triumphs.

SY: On the 7th I went up, and the staff was very happy to see me because they knew I had started the semester and was going to take care of Mrs. Abel. They said that Mrs. Abel was about the same; that she was crying and demanding although she was being less ritualistic. They explained this on the basis that she was lethargic. Her respirations were depressed to where the morphine had to be withheld if they were less than 10 per minute. The nurses told her they could not give her the narcotics if the respirations were depressed, so Mrs. Abel thought her respirations were being counted rather rapidly. There were some episodes during the previous week where they had to withhold the morphine and the patient would cry and carry on. Anyway, I said that I thought this was a terrible situation and what could be done about it? The nurses shrugged their shoulders. "Well what can you do about it." Then I said, "Well she doesn't focus so much on pain when you are in the room," and they said, "Oh, yes, we know that, but we just can't be in the room every minute," and they just refused to discuss it any further, and I certainly wasn't going to push it.

Anyway, I talked to the patient and told her that I was coming in to shampoo her hair, and she again wept about the uselessness of it all, which was to be the pattern of discussion for the ensuing weeks. The other thing is that I told the nursing staff that I was going to shampoo the hair, and they were pleased with this because she was pestering the staff about washing it.

SA: This was when you told me definitely that Dr. Colp was only coming when the evening staff was on, to see them and that communication between him and the day staff had completely disintegrated over his telling the patient one thing and the girls another.

SY: Yes, he was beginning to visit in the evenings because he didn't have to meet the day staff who had talked the loudest about getting the patient out.

SY: I saw Miss Lyon, the supervisor on the 9th. She opened the discussion by thanking me for taking care of Mrs. Abel and it was a tremendous relief for the staff to have me come in for two mornings a week because Mrs. Abel was so impossible. That's about all that related to this patient that we talked about.

SA: I had tried to see Miss Lyon prior to Christmas vacation but as there was a number of supervisors ill, I just couldn't catch up with her. She was never around. She just couldn't see me during that time, so we made arrangements to meet the first week after the new year, when everybody would be back and things were settled. I saw her then and she said that she was just as frustrated as everybody else. She didn't know what to do either. "I've been trying to spend some time in the floor in order to give the girls some relief." She was very much concerned about the staff. "We have been rotating then, but on the night shift there is only the night nurse and the aide and there is no way I can rotate them." The evening girls only had two nurses. She discussed the possibility of putting a float nurse on the floor, sort of as a special nurse for Mrs. Abel but, "It isn't fair to them nor is it fair to Mrs. Abel. . . . I'm really more concerned about my staff than I am about Mrs. Abel." And anyhow you would have a constant changing of personnel for Mrs. Abel with whom she would be unable to make a relationship, so it wasn't fair to Mrs. Abel. But the supervisor couldn't tolerate the thought of using a float—she might even lose her floats because they couldn't stand Mrs. Abel. Also she had been afraid that Mrs. Abel would die before Christmas and that then the girls would always feel guilty because they did not have a chance to resolve working through their feelings.

AS: We were concerned about this too—not that she would die, but die all of a sudden. . . .

SA: Right, because you had already said to me the best thing that could have happened for this woman was to die suddenly. In fact, that was the day that we told Shizu that if Mrs. Abel died right then and there she would be much better off—but that this would be horrible for the staff. And essentially, without my even suggesting it, Miss Lyon told me the same thing. She said that Dr. Colp was giving them very little support—"We just can't talk to him, we can't get to him." And she said, "When Dr. Tree finished his research, then we just have to get her out of here." And she said, "My last resort is the float nurse." You and I had been wondering whether they would ever put on extra nurses to special this woman. Would they go so far or had they considered transferring her to other floors. Because Elaine and the girls were already suggesting Mrs. Abel would be better off with a new staff and a new floor situation. The supervisor felt that Mrs. Abel needed continued support but really didn't know what to do about Mrs. Abel either. She is one of the first who really said that it is difficult to know how much pain Mrs. Abel is having. That's when she told me about Mrs. Abel losing the notebook. It was the day Mrs. Abel lost the notebook, and Miss Lyon was the first who told me about it. She said they were unable to find it. "I looked all over the place for it, because things will be in a real uproar up there." She also said she was glad to talk to me or Shizu (she had seen Shizu that morning) in planning what could be done for this woman. She was looking for me for some helpful advice which I still couldn't give her. . . .

SY: On January 8, the night nurse reported that Mrs. Abel cried during the night as if her heart were breaking and she said, "I want someone to love me." Discussing the incident later, the nurse said that what happened was the patient reached out to her and she instinctively moved away from the patient, and this is when the patient said, "I want somebody to love me."

AS: This is the first time that we know of that the patient has said anything like this directly rather than by all the other oblique ways that she had been using. Right?

SY: Yes. Then the night nurse said that she realized what was happening so she took Mrs. Abel in her arms and let her cry. She described the crying as something different from the crying in the past. It was the crying of real despair. She said, "You know, I felt so terrible I felt like crying, too." I said that maybe it was a good thing that the patient got it out, and it was probably a good thing that she did let her cry. The night nurse, by the way, is a young nurse, runs around with some kids in the Master's program and is more oriented to a psychological approach.

Mrs. Abel was sleeping very soundly when I went into her room. The narcotics were due but I didn't wake her. I held off for about half an hour. Actually the patient didn't become aware that I had held off until about 30 minutes after I gave the injection. When she got to writing it down, she said, "You know I can't stand the

118

pain if it is not on time." She cried quite a bit about the pain, and I told her I was sorry I didn't give it to her on time and the next time I would wake her up. Then I immediately changed the discussion to the shampoo because I couldn't tolerate this discussion on pain. Discussion on pain then stopped because we were talking about pleasant things.

AS: Did you feel negligent about the timing?

SY: I debated about waking her up and finally decided I'd better do it or be in a hassle for the rest of the morning. You know, you feel like a dirty dog if she is snoring away and then you wake her up. I got a feeling of what the night nurses were probably going through.

On the 9th, the following day, periodically the patient would say, "I want to be in a coma." Then she would say, "This is terrible, I wish I could go in my sleep and die in my sleep." She kept saying this periodically throughout the morning.

AS: What are you doing when she is saying this?

SY: I'm listening, I'm nodding my head, I'm encouraging her to talk or I would say, "Do you really want to be in a coma?" But she would never go beyond this. She would keep on saying she wanted to be in a coma. Then she would cry out very loudly, "Please God do something, either take me or make me better. I can't stand it." It would be very loud and this would be interspersed with, "I want to die, I want to be in coma." Apparently this had been going on for about a week prior to my taking care of her. Then at one point: "I don't want to be a baby but I can't help it. I know it annoys the nurse (crying)." I said, "Do you think it annoys the nurse?" She said yes, the nurses tell her that if she cries she just makes herself more upset. Then I asked if crying helped her. She said that she had to get it out, the only thing she got any relief from was from crying. So I told her to go ahead and cry.

AS: I get a sense that she was at her most lucid, more than on all the many days that we have talked about previously. Now for the first time she sounds like she is aware of what she is doing to the nurses; she sounds like she knows she is reaching out for something; she is appealing directly and very forcefully and very rationally to God. She is not really talking to you so much but talking with great rationality—whereas everything else you have said before sounds like most of her talking was very oblique. Though she may have known many things, she was not saying it to the outside world Do you agree with this?

119

SA: Yes.

SY: For two weeks it was a loud "please God," and then about two weeks before the very end she would be muttering to herself and I would say, "What are you saying?" and she would say, "I'm praying." She didn't need to say it out loud.

AS: So that she herself is "instinctively" in a new phase of dying. Yet outside the room nurses are talking as if it is the same old behavior. They are saying there is no great changes. Is that correct?

SA: Yes.

SY: Yes. . . . I washed the patient's hair and this time she didn't give me the great detailed instruction. She let me put up her hair any way I wanted. She completely complied with whatever I did.

AS: What exactly were the nurses then writing on the charts? Any indication that they caught this new phase in her behavior?

SY: They described that she was praying a lot, was less alert. That was about all. They described her as being less ritualistic.

SA: But they never did describe her as less complaining.

AS: So they are responding to changes of certain kinds. But that doesn't mean they are spending more time with her.

SY: No.

AS: When they say she is praying, are they aware that she is making her peace with the world—which is what I assume she is doing.

SY: No.

SA: That never even occurred to me.

AS: If she is not making her peace, she is at least preparing for the passage that she knows (and wishes because of the pain) is coming.

SA: She hadn't accepted it yet though, because when I talked to her later on, the 13th, she said, "If I am dying, if there is nothing more they can do for me, then I will accept a lobotomy; but if there is, then I don't want anything to do with a lobotomy."

AS: I think we can assume she never really, strictly speaking, made her peace. Right down to the very end when she says, "Let me die on the table," she was still vacillating. But my point is that now she is willing to consider really full face and realistically the alternatives: either cure me or get rid of me.

120

SA: These are the alternatives, but there is a point at which there was a decided change—about half way following after January 13—when various nurses pick up the "change in personality."

AS: Is there less insistence after the January 6th shampoo by her in terms of the body itself—less attention to her body?

SY: That's right.

AS: Does she let herself go in appearance at all?

SY: Not entirely.

AS: I'm thinking now in terms of her hair, her manicure.

SY: No. That never went.

SA: That never went. The chaplain felt that she was taking even less care at the end about whether her garments covered herself; but her appearance, her makeup, always stayed the same.

SY: The aide, for example gave Mrs. Abel credit for being aware of her appearance.

During the hair setting she asked for a lot of things. I would be right in the middle of putting the hair up and then she would ask me for a kleenex. She would want it right then and there and I would say, "Just a minute and I will get it for you," and she would press me to do it immediately. About the fourth interference I was getting a little irritated so I told her that I found it very irritating; she knew that I would do these things for her as soon as I could and that I only had two hands, and that I didn't like it when she would do these things. Then she began crying and said, "Please don't hate me." I told her I didn't hate her but this irritated me when she did this, and she said she didn't want to irritate me and I thought, "My God, she is just like a child," so I thought: I can't do any more when I am irritated. I will get madder and madder and I won't be able to tolerate her any more. The patient was less talkative; her physical condition was very poor; her feet were very swollen and her arms looked terrible. I noticed, too, that the patient's marking down of narcotics in her book was less elaborate. She used blue ink both for the writing down and the crossing out. She stated that she realized that the new hormones were not helping her. She had hoped that this would stop the pain process and that Dr. Tree was starting these new drug studies on her, but she had not seen him.

AS: Were you struck by the change in her psychological bearing on this day?

SY: Yes. She was really talking about death very differently.

AS: We understand now there was a great change on this day. I'm asking you if then you realized it? Did it show up in your notes?

SA: I think it's coming through in the flavor of her words. Before when Mrs. Abel cried and talked about dying you felt very inadequate, very depressed, very incompetent. Here Shizu is saying, "I felt this was working, this was effective for Mrs. Abel. She was able to cry and I let her cry, feeling that this was good for her." I don't catch now your feeling of total inadequacy in this situation. Yet only half an hour ago your tonal quality reflected sheer inability to cope with Mrs. Abel. Now a sort of sadness is coming through in your voice.

SY: On that day I taped my notes and a friend who came to visit said, "God, you sound like a funeral." And I answered, "Well, it's pretty soon."

The team leader said I deserved a gold medal for taking care of Mrs. Abel, and I asked what do you mean? "Well you deserve a gold medal for putting up with her." Then I said that I thought Mrs. Abel was teaching me a great deal about dying patients and that I hoped whatever I did was a help. She said it sure helped them because it gave them a breather. Then I said that of course I don't see the patient twenty-four hours a day so it makes a difference in how much of her I can tolerate. Then she said well they didn't know, but I sure deserved a gold medal.

AS: There were two phases preceding this general reaction. First, when you came on the ward the personnel were very happy to have you there taking this troublesome patient off their hands. Then they reacted against you because you were all tied up with the whole business of pain. Then when you came back on the floor after a week or so of absence she was then clearly terminal and in a "nothing more to do" phase, and they were very happy to have you there again until she died. Am I right?

SY: Yes and they had one less person to assign to the patient.

SA: But you still felt fairly isolated from them. Right up to the end you felt that only you and the social worker were able to communicate with one another. You were both sort of isolated on the floor. Yet, possibly because you took off for a couple of weeks, they had all they could take, and they wanted you back.

The other thing that I notice in the sound of your voice is your response to the staff about what they were doing. Your voice reflects that you were now out of the critical stage of criticizing the staff for their inability to take care of this patient. That was either because

122

of the work that you had done in the fieldwork class or because the three of us had been discussing what had been happening among the staff. It's in here that you really begin to pick up and use a different frame of reference than only your nursing frame of reference.

SY: On January 9, the head nurse stated that Mrs. Abel seemed happier and quieter and thought perhaps it was the shampoo and set, because everybody had been complimenting the patient and telling her how nice she looked. Mrs. Abel was more alert that day. We discussed her care and decided that probably a manicure could be fitted in. After I gave the first injection, I looked for the narcotic book that she marks up but I couldn't locate it. I thought, "Horrors Mrs. Abel will fall apart—the security blanket, you know, what am I going to do?" I searched the room and I couldn't find it. Knowing how she felt about the book, I asked if she had another book in which she could record the medications. She said she did. I said "fine" and thought I would go out and let everybody know and alert them to this book—partly because I wanted to know what would happen. They were on rounds. I stopped the head nurse and said in a half whisper, "I can't find the book." She smiled and five minutes later when I stopped people and asked them, everybody knew, including the janitor, that Mrs. Abel had lost this book. There was considerable merriment about it and they said things like, "Are you sure you didn't throw it away?" or "Maybe it's a good thing." Anyway I said, "You people are terrible, you know she is going to find another book anyway." Elizabeth, I think, said, "Yes that's true, she will probably find a new book anyway." (It kind of reminded me that the staff was acting like Lucy with Peanuts depriving Linus of his security blanket.) The assistant head nurse, who seemed particularly amused by this incident, said, "You know, I just have to see this"! She went to the patient's room. When I went in there the patient was *very calmly* saying to the assistant head nurse that she hated to lose the pen because it was brand new. You know, I felt ugly enough to enjoy the fact that the patient was pretty calm in the situation. Anyway, fortunately I found the book. It had dropped in the wastebasket, and I hadn't dug down deep enough.

SA: Miss Lyon told me about the book. Then I didn't find out what the final outcome was until Shizu filled me in.

SY: I was particularly amused when Miss Lyon got in the act, too. I didn't think it would go this far.

SA: When I saw the supervisor she was drastically concerned about this. She thought this was a "catastrophe."

SY: Anyway, the patient had periods of crying that day but she didn't seem to cry as often. She would pray at times, loudly again. Then she talked about her father at great length, indicating she was very fond of him. At one point she said she used to enjoy playing the piano and singing and thought she had a pretty good voice. She talked about liking opera and how much she liked Madame Butterfly.

AS: Is this the first time she was talking about the past not in a ritualistic fashion but in a reviewing, remembering kind of mood?

SY: Yes.

AS: This is one of the signs that people are preparing for death. That is why I asked.

SY: Then she talked about enjoying Madame Butterfly's "One Fine Day" and sang a couple of bars of that—and started to cry. I asked her what was the matter and she said, "Oh, Shizu, I don't want to die." I said it must be very hard for you to take, and that I wished I could help her. She cried for quite a period and I just felt terrible. Then she fell into a doze and later woke up with a very pained expression on her face. I asked her what happened. She had a bad dream about the frustration of buying a house. Then she remarked that her dreams always had the same theme—one of frustration—and she felt this was the pattern of her life: she was thwarted in pursuing art; her marriage was bad, and her marriage previous to that was bad; and now she had this terrible illness. She dwelt on this at great length.

I asked if she had seen the social worker. She had but she didn't want to pursue it. I thought there was no sense in trying to find out what the discharge plans were; I didn't think there was going to be one anyway. At the end of the morning June and Helen thought it was a good idea I had washed the patient's hair—the first time they discussed her in terms of body image, and the relationship of pain to body image. They brought up Mrs. Abel's discussion of her photograph. I thought it strange that this was the first type of objective discussion I had had.

SY: I saw the chaplain the same morning. As a last resort, he had raised the question to Mrs. Abel that perhaps she should take the attitude of a courageous woman facing death. But he didn't think it helped her. Also, with me he questioned whether there should not be a team conference so that the nurses could bring out their guilt feelings and hostile feelings. I didn't push this, and he never did it.

AS: It sounds as if now that the patient is clearly signaling in a rather realistic way her thoughts about dying, the chaplain is now able to pick up these signals and say, "You will have to be courageous." It also sounds as if he is getting prepared himself against her dying soon or suddenly.

SY: There is another important point. On January 8, Dr. Colp made a notation: "Dr. Tree plans pain research. Discharge patient after that." He put that in the chart.

AS: Did he believe it?

SA: I don't think so. Dr. Tree never appeared after the first of the year, because it's then that they start talking about the lobotomy. Tree had already pulled out before the discussion of lobotomy, according to Tree's secretary, simply because Mrs. Abel was going to be discharged. There were no more funds.

SY: On January 10, I met the social worker who stated that plans had been made for Mrs. Abel's discharge from the hospital to a nursing home in Contra Costa County, following the pain study by Dr. Tree. The patient would be on aid to the totally disabled, therefore would not be a financial drain on the household and there was no lien on the house. The social worker had been seeing the patient regularly about twice a week. She felt that Dr. Colp seemed to have considerable anxiety about discharging the patient, and had made a very strange statement that he felt better about discharging Mrs. Abel now as he felt the hospital had repaid Mrs. Abel for her services as a research subject. The social worker spent some time reassuring Dr. Colp that the patient actually had been carried for a long period and that facilities where she was going seemed adequate. She was struck by his "repaying" explanation.

AS: Is this social worker trained as a psychiatric social worker?

SY: She's a medical social worker who is working on her Master's degree. Yes, she does use the language, the vocabulary of a psychiatric social worker?

SA: On the 13th of January I was walking through the clinic section of the hospital. I practically walked by Mrs. Abel. She was sitting in a wheelchair outside the EEG Department. She looked very, very pale; I hadn't seen her since Christmas when I pulled out, and she was so pale, so white, that I thought, "My God." She started to cry, "They are going to do a lobotomy. I heard that makes a vegetable out of you." She wanted to know what I thought of a lobotomy and whether she would become a vegetable if they did one. Then she said, "They can't do anything about my arm because I've been in pain all night; they can't give me relief. I cried for an hour this morning and still couldn't get anything. If they can't do anything about my arm, if they can't cure me then I'll let them do the lobotomy. But if they can do something for me, then I don't want anything to do with this lobotomy." This was the first I heard of the possibility of a lobotomy, other than Dr. Colp having said there was nothing more that they can really do for her *but* the lobotomy. Mrs. Abel said, "I just can't stand this pain any longer." She constantly referred to the pain.

She was asking questions of me; she wanted to know *my* opinion on a lobotomy. I frankly had no experience in taking care of post-op lobotomy patients and what I knew was from hearsay. I couldn't give her any first-hand information other than that I didn't think she would be a vegetable and ask her if she had talked further with the physician, what they had said about the lobotomy, and so forth.

AS: You came through like a real staff nurse.

SA: Right. Very much so. Then I talked to Shizu and asked if she knew anything about it, or what had Mrs. Abel been like.

SY: On January 13 I had heard about this so I went up to see the patient. In fact, I was startled by this information about lobotomy because I hadn't ever heard it being used for this situation. I thought it was a pretty terrible thing to do to Mrs. Abel, colored by my own experience with lobotomized patients. I was filled with the frustration of having to restrain some of these *adult* patients to toilet train—this kind of thing—and it just filled me with great agitation. Anyway, I asked the staff nurses what the lobotomy was about and they just shrugged their shoulders. They just didn't know what was going on. They didn't seem to want to discuss it. When I saw the patient she stated that Dr. Colp had posed the possibility of a lobotomy as a means of controlling pain and that she was waiting the arrival of the neurologist. She said that the information from Dr. Colp was more on the favorable side because he was for the procedure, and felt that it was a very biased opinion. She had read, however, that the lobotomy left the patient like a vegetable, so she wasn't sure that she wanted this, but at the same time she just couldn't tolerate the pain any longer.

Mrs. Abel flipped back and forth on this, and said if her condition was a matter of six months, or a year or so, then she would have the lobotomy done because she could not stand the pain any longer. But if it was a matter of four or five years, she said, "Suppose they find a cure for cancer?"—then she wouldn't be alert to enjoy life.

I told the chaplain that I thought she seemed disturbed and would he please come to see her. He said, "I certainly will go to see her—

126

today if I possibly can. If not, tomorrow night." He was very disturbed by it. He said, "Are you *sure* it's not a cordotomy?"

SA: And for good reasons. He had worked in mental hospitals for quite a while and he had seen a number of lobotomized patients who were, as far as he was concerned, a bunch of vegetbles, who had no ability left to do anything at all. They were unable to make any decisions. They were so lethargic they couldn't do anything. He said, "I just don't know about these lobotomies." He was very upset about even its possibility and did not really seem in favor of Mrs. Abel having a lobotomy, in spite of the fact that she was in a lot of pain and the amount of medication she was on made her lethargic anyway—she wasn't functioning. But he was terribly opposed to the procedure.

SY: Later Mrs. Abel pressed me for an opinion. "What do you think I should do?" I said, "Do you want to know what I think?" She asked, "Have you ever seen a lobotomy used for my type of case?" I answered that I had not and she said, "I wish you had seen a patient where it was done for my problem." She kept saying this and, "Then you could help me decide what to do." I told her I couldn't give her any answers because I hadn't seen one. She was anxiously awaiting the arrival of the neurologist for further discussion of this procedure, and I asked her to continue it with the neurologist. I really felt cornered. I knew that she knew that I was being evasive about this thing.

SA: Dr. Colp was away at a convention, so he wasn't available to either us or the patient.

SY: Did you see . . . .

SA: No, as a matter of fact, that's the last time I saw Mrs. Abel—on January 13.

SY: On January 15, I went up to see her and she was at X-ray for a skull study. I ran into Miss Sadina, the regular social worker asigned to the unit. We went into a discussion of Mrs. Abel, and she made the statement that Dr. Colp had tremendous difficulty in discharging his patients from the hospital, and that this had been their experience with him before, and that she had warned the social worker that there was this possibility. Then she became quite disturbed when I began to tell her all that had happened. She hadn't realized that is was as messy as the story was beginning to become.

SA: She had been on the floor a couple of times.

SY: She is concerned with discharge plans for other patients. Apparently the young social worker is working with the supervisor and doesn't discuss the case with Miss Sadina.

When I asked the assistant head nurse, Elaine, what was going on about the lobotomy and what it was all about, and did she know anything about it, she shook her head in great dismay. "You know, I just don't know, I just don't know." She added that she recently read a book by Frank Slaughter on lobotomized patients and what she read was a pretty dismal and terrible story. "You know, I just don't know. It seems like a horrible idea." Previous discussions with this nurse have always been real animated, loud, almost what amounted to hatred being expressed about this patient. But this was a very subdued, very thoughtful discussion. I got the impression that she would rather tolerate this patient, as horrible as she was, rather than have her go through this procedure. By the way, the notation made on that day by the physician was, "If procedure not done, discharge home in a few weeks."

SA: You had been talking to some of the nurses and had now found that some of the individual nurses would admit to you that she was following Mrs. Abel's routine but might not admit this to June. You were finding this separately amongst each of the staff involved.

SY: Yes, they were going along with the gag individually.

The following day I found the patient sleeping soundly. I called her several times but couldn't rouse her. The nursing staff again said they just didn't know about this lobotomy. They weren't sure if it was the answer to Mrs. Abel's problem. There was a general, subdued, disturbed discussion about this procedure.

Then on January 21, when I saw the patient, she was talking to the social worker. Shortly after I arrived the social worker walked away, and Mrs. Abel looked at her and said, "Shizu, how I envy people who can walk," and she cried for a period. When I asked about the surgery, she just couldn't decide what was the right thing to do, and again talked about the decision being in terms of how long she was to live. Again I asked her if the decision was entirely up to her and what did she think she needed to know? She said the decision was left up to her and that her husband told her she should do what she thought was right. When asking her what she felt she needed to know, and in trying to find out what Dr. Colp had told her about a time limit, I asked her several different ways. She never answered, she skirted the subject. She was told by the neurologist that the lobotomy would not stop the pain directly but that it would lessen the anxiety and, therefore, relieve the pain. So she emphasized over and over that the pain was *real* and that it was not from her mind. She was also told that she would be less alert and things wouldn't bother her as much.

Then she said, "You know, Shiz, that I am deformed." I thought it was interesting that this was the first time that she had ever used the word "deformed," because in previous discussions she had always changed the subject or always gone on to her talk about disillusionment, or she is sensitive to beauty and all that sort of stuff. Anyway, she said, "Because I am deformed, in order to compensate, I have used my mind and developed my mind; I'm not brilliant, but I have used it, and I have developed it to the optimum. I have always prided myself on having a brain, and I don't want—I don't know if I want to be less aware of what's going on." She continued "At the same time, I can't take any more pain."

We discussed it at some length, and I was thinking: My God, this is the only thing that this poor woman has left—the thing that she in her own self image was a good brain even though she was deformed. What are we going to do with this woman? Do we take this away, too? I was really in a quandry about—I mean why she would have so much indecision. I told her that I felt the decision was a real difficult one and was there anything that I might help her with, or anyone that I might talk with about her? Again she didn't push this.

After this discussion she said, "I wonder what it feels like to die, I wonder what it feels like to die." She then went into a discussion about her sister dying at the age of thirty from TB. I said that her sister was young and asked if she was with her sister when she died? The sister died in a sanatorium and she wasn't with her. Mrs. Abel went on to say that her sister was a very, very beautiful and very, very sophisticated girl and had lots and lots of boyfriends and that she, on the other hand, was very shy and very bookish and didn't go out with men until well in her twenties. Other things she said made me feel that there was always a certain degree of jealousy about her sister. I wondered as I listened to her whether there were death wishes involved and whether these were making her feel guilty. She kept saying, "I wonder what it feels like to die." I asked if she thought about this a great deal. All she answered was, "I wonder, I wonder," almost as if talking to herself.

Then there was a long silence, and she asked. "After I get home from the nursing home will you visit me?" I asked if she wanted me to. "Yes, Shizu, you know we could go on long drives together," and she went on and the story became very disconnected; she had a faraway look in her eyes as if daydreaming about all the places she would visit, and all the things we could do together. This went on for some time. Then I said, "Do you think you will be able to drive your car again?" She looked at me and said, "Shizu, I know

I am daydreaming; I know I am not going to be able to drive again. I know I am going to die." Then she cried and said, "This is terrible, I never thought I would be this way." I must have sat with her for fifteen minutes or so while she cried. There was nothing I could do except to sit with her and let her cry. Then after she stopped crying I told her I was in the midst of finals and that I would visit her as soon as they were over. She said how she envied me; how much she had enjoyed school and had been an honor student throughout high school. Then we talked for some time about the pleasant times she had in high school and the courses she had liked, and so on.

Then on the 15th, in looking over the patient's chart, I noticed: "Discharge patient if not surgery." The notation for January 16: "If neurosurgery successful, discharge home eight to ten days following." In the interim period that I hadn't seen her, the patient's morphine dosage had been decreased to 16 milligrams (previously 20 milligrams) because the respirations were becoming more depressed. The order also read, "Withhold morphine for one hour if the respirations are less than ten." Several episodes were noted where the patient became very upset because the drugs were withheld. The nurses' notes continued to describe the patient as being weepy, demanding, and very difficult to manage.

AS: Did Mrs. Abel know why the morphine was being withheld?

SY: Yes, she knew this from the very beginning, back in the latter part of December when this was taking place. There was this *tremendous* ruckus going on! It was after Christmas holidays, and it was during the Christmas week that she was having such a terrible time with the narcotics.

AS: What did the respiration phenomenon mean to her?

SY: Apparently it didn't mean that much to her because she said —she used to pant rapidly.

SA: Shizu, you came to me with a funny story about how ridiculous that was. Here this woman was hyperventilating to prove that she was alright so that the staff would give her the medication. Mrs. Abel didn't have a full awareness of what decreased respirations meant in connection with death.

AS: What does it mean?

SA: Well if she had had too much more morphine, she actually would have died from an overdose of toxicity in morphine. For people they get to in time, the antidote saves them. The drug that can be used there is an antidote for morphine toxicity, but Mrs. Abel had a tremendous backlog or treatment doses of morphine. But she just wasn't aware of this.

AS: What did the respiration phenomenon mean to her? Have you any idea? They must have presented her with an alternative—that they had to do this because. . . .

SA: Because her respirations were decreased. They would count them and if her respirations were more than ten, no more than fourteen I think . . .

SY: Yes, early in December it was more than fourteen.

SA: Yes, if it was more than fourteen she could have it—so she would pant in order to prove that her respirations had not slowed down.

AS: Did the nurses recognize this as fraudulent?

SA: The night nurses did because they were counting the respirations at night while she was asleep.

SY: This is when they picked it up. The patient never questioned me or wanted to know why it was withheld. The point that she kept discussing was, "The nurses keep saying I want to count your respiration when actually what they mean is respirations." She would dwell on this every time I would go in, respirations versus respiration.

AS: That illustrates lay versus relatively technical words. At the same time, I suppose they couldn't say, "You might pass out entirely." They probably never made the connection for her between death and the morphine.

SY: She never asked either, because I was waiting for her to ask. And I never told her because she never asked. I thought afterwards, suppose she had asked? How would I explain it to her? I think I would have kept her distracted by talking and being with her.

SA: In other words, not give her the information?

SY: I don't know what I would do.

SA: Why not? *Why not tell her:* "Look there is a possibility you could have an overdose of morphine." What would have been *so* wrong about telling Mrs. Abel?

SY: Oh, I don't think I would have . . . .

SA: You would tell her about any other drug.

SY: That's true.

SA: If somebody asks, "Can I dies from this, or what would happen to me if I had too much of this?" you tell them the toxicity. In fact, then patients will tell you, you know, that sometimes they develop the symptoms of the toxicity occasionally, like ringing of ears from aspirins.

SY: Now it was January 24 and things were status quo. The neurologists had seen Mrs. Abel several times and notes indicated that they believed her a good candidate for surgery—a lobotomy. The surgery was withheld because of instrument repairs and also because Dr. Colp was out of town.

AS: If the instruments had been ready, they might have done a lobotomy then, unless another decision had been made?

SY: Yes. They were still discussing pro and con.

SA: And these were special instruments. I had never heard of them before — they were stereotaxic. They were not customary surgical instruments which you would use on a routine lobotomy.

SY: Again the patient was battling back and forth about this. Though she had been discussing it with the neurologist and was half way in agreement, she was still in great indecision, and she was questioning everybody.

SA: I think this is why she hit me and asked me these questions originally, because she hadn't seen me for a month.

SY: Again she pressed me for an opinion, and she remarked, "You sound doubtful." I said, "I do?" And she said, "Yes, you keep asking me all these questions." I answered that I wanted to see how she felt about it. I knew she was cornered, and I was cornered. I found it interesting that she was very, very alert to the feelings of the people around her and their indecision. My last patient, too, had picked up my anxiety about his discharge, as well as the resident's. That patient picked it up right away and kept saying I sounded doubtful. I found it interesting that this patient did the same thing.

SA: You also felt that she was picking up anxiety about the operation from the chaplain and the social worker.

SY: Yes. The social worker, too, when I stopped her, said the patient had picked up the anxiety and said to her, "You sound doubtful. To me, Mrs. Abel had complained before about the staff but this time she was very, very loud and bitter, saying that they were very short tempered with her, and were not answering the light, making her wait for long periods, etc. She went on at great and unusual length. When I asked the staff how they felt about Mrs. Abel's surgery, they said the patient was the same as usual—indicating bad as usual—and they didn't want to discuss the surgery with me. But I didn't get the concern of the prior week; that they thought it was bad. Somehow they didn't want to discuss it with the same kind of personal concern I had noticed the week before.

AS: They had made up their minds that it was bad, and knew it might be done now.

SY: Yes, they knew that it was imminent. It was already scheduled. It was being withheld because of surgical repairs. It did not make sense, but they were resigned to whatever decision was made. On January 25, the notation said, "Dr. Abram has seen the patient and plans surgery." But there was nothing on the notation about whether it was to be a hypophysectomy or otherwise.

On February 4, I ran into the social worker who stated that the patient was talking about a hypophysectomy instead of a lobotomy. Did I know anything about it? I didn't know. All I knew about a hypophysectomy was in reference to tumors. She said the patient had been told by the neurologist that the surgery was to stop the pain. I went by to see the patient again, and she was sleeping soundly. I called her several times and couldn't awaken her. The nurse's notes on February 4 indicate that the patient was getting more and more lethargic.

On February 7 I hadn't seen the patient for some days and during the interim period—well, on January 27, Dr. Colp had made the statement that "both myself and the nurses have noted a personality change in the patient," and that it was an odd kind of behavior and she had temper tantrums. Also, the patient was not responding to diuretics, and he felt that this was due partially to the estrogens that the patient was on and so more drugs were given to increase the diuresis. The patient was complaining of tightness in the chest and the throat. The nurse's notes indicated increased irritability and weeping in between lethargy and such statements were made by the patient as, " I want to die." "Please help me." And, "Please God help me." The nurse's notes also indicated that the patient was very upset, screaming—sort of tantrum behavior.

AS: Did they also use the words "changed personality"?

SY: No.

SA: They must have said something because when I talked to Dr. Colp his wording was, "The nurses tell me that she has had a

133

change of personality." That's when I began to push to see if the change of personality meant that Mrs. Abel had finally decided she was now dying. I am pretty sure those are the words they used because Dr. Colp sort of repeated them as the nurses had said, "We noted a change the other day."

SY: On February 5 the doctor's notes indicate, "The patient's respirations are becoming more and more depressed." And the morphine sulphate order was changed to 12 milligrams instead of the previous 16 milligrams.

SA: Thus it dropped from 24 to 16 down to 12.

SY: Yes, and the patient is less alert and has times of incompetence. After the semester break, on February 10, I saw Dr. Colp on the ward. "Oh, I see you are back from semester break." He had just seen Mrs. Abel and said that I would have to go in to see her.

SA: I also talked with Dr. Colp on February 10 to find out what had been going on. He said, "You know, I am not as interested in this case as you are. I'm not taking this problem home with me anymore. Mrs. Abel is the only patient I have on the floor, and you are more interested in this person than I am." My thought was, "That's what you think, you are not taking it home"!

Anyway, the lobotomy had been postponed for two weeks because of the instruments, and now they were to do a hypophysectomy. He said, "It's my experience that it only works for the people who have had regression of tumor when they were on hormonal therapy (which Mrs. Abel was on). Since she has no regression of tumor there is no hormone that will work for her. I only expect the possibility of 10% improvement with the surgical procedure." He added, "It isn't done for pain but for reduction of tumor." I baited him with my knowledge and brief experience nursing a hypophysectomy patient who had had dramatic pain relief. He said this is possible but really rather secondary, and that a hypophysectomy is what the neurosurgeons wanted to do and it was their decision. He remarked that Dr. Tree was *not* going to do any research on Mrs. Abel but didn't indicate any reason why Dr. Tree had changed his mind. Also, he said, "I was going to discharge her about a month ago but when they decided to do the lobotomy I held off." I wanted to know what kind of arrangements had been made, and that's when he told about the arrangements with the Contra Costa Hospital and the nursing home; then he went on to tell about Mr. Abel's fluctuating bank account and that this would really take a toll on the family savings —and this just wasn't fair. He elaborated at great length. On this day, he also told me that a week previous the nurses noted a personality change in Mrs. Abel. (I thought then that possibly she accepted the fact that death was now imminent and inevitable.) He said, "She is gradually losing hope, and I don't give her any hope."

He was beginning gradually to decrease the medication. "I am thinking about cutting it about 7 milligrams at a time." When he said, "When the nurses started checking her respiration, they were down below 10," I thought: these girls are good nurses, they have been checking the respiration. This is a routine procedure and certainly if they were giving massive doses of narcotics they would be checking the respiration. (I am assuming you were, Shizu.) But his implication was that when the nurses finally got around to checking, the respirations were already below 10, therefore I (Dr. Colp) had to start cutting the medication. It's as if the nurses were behind.

He said, "I am still cutting it 5 milligrams a week because her respirations are still dropping at night." (They were checking her respirations at night while she was asleep.) He said she didn't need it any more. (In fact, Mrs. Abel never knew they were cutting the amount.) "This just goes to prove that her pain was mostly anxiety and not physiological pain." As far as he was concerned, it was not lack of alertness on Mrs. Abel's part because of her terminal state.

AS: But he is not saying that she didn't feel a thing.

SA: That's right. Later on in another discussion he very clearly said that although she used the word "tightness" and so forth, and is very anxious about it, I, too, if I had been in her place might describe this as pain. It was very real to Mrs. Abel as far as he was concerned.

SA: He again asked me what I was going to do with all this information. I fed him a few tidbits about these are things we have learned and these will be good for nursing care and planning. He was interested in what we were learning; what we were going to do with this material. I really had to prove to him again that I was doing research.

He then remarked that Mrs. Abel was the only patient that he had on the 12th Floor, and he was not going to admit any more. This was the first time I became aware that because of Mrs. Abel he was now never going to admit another patient to the 12th Floor. That's what he said on the 10th. (Later he told me there would be a few patients he would admit for terminal care for a two or three day period, but he would at least never admit anyone for as lengthy a stay or Mrs. Abel's.) But on that earlier day he wasn't *ever* going to admit anybody, period! Also he was going to do nothing but research. He went on to say that the people above him gave free rein to do whatever he wanted to, and the only reason he had ever admitted patients to the hospital was because the man preceding him on the fellowship had done so. So he was following in that pattern. But his superiors were not questioning what he was doing, and he could spend all his time on research and this was what he was going to do. "It just isn't fair to use the budget of surgery nor is it fair to use their bed space."

AS: I remember that you came rushing, all excited and flustered and fluttery about this. We had earlier predicated that, "We can't tell what will happen as this drama unfolds." But we expected Mrs. Abel to become comatose in some weeks and then it would end. We were taken aback by the precise procedure that they decided upon but more astonished to see the drama break wide open all over again. It was as if another chapter was now about to be written when we thought the story was about closed.

SA: This meant also opening another chapter for the girls on the ward, who had essentially closed it thinking that the patient was going to die on the floor. ("We don't have any hope of getting rid of her.") And now again there was this possibility that Mrs. Abel would undergo surgery and then leave the floor. This would be their way of getting rid of Mrs. Abel. So it reopened that chapter as well.

AS: We thought we were studying a terminal patient and now we again were dealing with a "pain patient." Even though both pain and death run side by side, pain was getting subdued with death coming on; but now the pain again came into great focus. As a matter of fact, that's why Shirley became a much more active observer again as Mrs. Abel approached her end.

SY: I will now continue my discussion with Dr. Colp. I think I ended by saying that he said I didn't have to go in and see the patient. I asked him why.

SA: This followed my discussion with him. He went immediately from me to see Mrs. Abel, and then you talked to him right afterwards.

SY: He said, "Well she is so depressing and she cries all the time." He didn't blame the nursing staff for spending so little time with her because she was so depressing. Sprinkled throughout the conversation was, "You really don't have to go in to see her." I was thinking, "My God, you feel so terrible about it you have to have everybody else sharing your feeling."

Anyway, I asked about the hypophysectomy and he said pretty much the same thing that Shirley had reported, and emphasized that the neurologist knew more about the situation than he did. I asked about her condition and could she risk it, and would there be other problems as a result of the hypophysectomy—in terms of her present electrolyte imbalance. He brushed it off. "Oh, we can replace that easy enough."

SA: That comes up afterwards when he emphasizes that he had been feeding her enough potassium so that electrolyte imbalance shouldn't be a problem.

SY: He seemed very anxious to terminate the discussion. I asked, "Will the patient be coming back on this unit?" He said the patient would more than likely go to the 7th Floor, and he felt that this was a good thing, as there would be new people, etc. Then, "Well, I have to run off to see another patient." As he left, "You know you really don't have to go in to see the patient." I felt he was projecting his own feelings.

SA: You felt also that he was really emphasizing them, because you commented to me that he not only said this once but several times.

SY: And he couldn't tolerate anybody who could half-way tolerate the patient.

To continue: When I went to see the patient I was shocked to find her so deteriorated. Her color was terrible . . . .

SA: This was the 10th of February. And the last time you had seen her was on the 24th of January?

SY: I saw her on February 4, but she was sleeping and I couldn't awaken her.

SA: This meant that you had come in during the semester break anyway to see Mrs. Abel.

SY: January 24 was the last time I really spent time talking to her. Anyway, on February 10 she looked terrible. There was swelling on the right angle of her jaw and further extension of cancer on the neck, which was quite visible. She stated that surgery was scheduled for the following day and that she was anxiously awaiting surgery because she just could not tolerate the pain anymore. She cried and said she never thought she would be like this. She wished she could die and she wept for a period. I felt terrible for her. I thought what a *horrible* way to die, in so much pain, distraught, and unloved. I stood at her bedside and she must have cried again for about fifteen minutes. All I could do was to hold her hand and let her cry because I knew there wasn't anything I could do to comfort her, and felt that she probably knew that I wanted to understand how she felt. Mrs. Abel again complained bitterly about the staff, that they were very, very short tempered with her.

The nursing staff stated that Mrs. Abel was less alert; she was having temper tantrums—when drugs were withheld she would get very, very upset and scream and holler. When they moved her rapidly she would scream out in pain and had "temper tantrums." When I stopped the head nurse and asked her what the surgery was all about and what was their understanding of the hypophysectomy, she said she didn't know what was going on: "I just haven't seen the neurologist." The laboratory was having difficulty getting blood from Mrs. Abel because of the antibody problem. She had been on so many drugs that there was a strange antibody reaction. They felt that possibly the patient would not be going to surgery the next day even though she was scheduled. When I said that I would be in to take care of her the following morning the head nurse said, "You know, you are very brave to take care of Mrs. Abel." I asked her what she meant. "Well you are brave for putting up with Mrs. Abel."

I wanted to push it further with her but she wouldn't go beyond this—I was very brave in putting up with her. On February 11, the following morning, I went up, halfway expecting the patient to go to surgery. The head nurse stated that Mrs. Abel would probably not go even though she was scheduled because blood was not available. When I asked how Mrs. Abel was doing, "Oh, the usual." When I went into the patient's room, the patient said, "My God, I'm so glad you are here, you know, like an angel from Heaven. Thank God, the other nurses are so short tempered." She said, "I will be so glad when the surgery is over with," because she couldn't stand the pain any longer. She repeated this several times, and *then* I realized nobody had told her that she was *not* going to surgery. What they were doing was saving this for me, because they knew that if they went in and announced this to her she would cry and carry on. They couldn't tolerate this.

AS: How did they know you were coming?

SY: I had told the head nurse that I was coming. That was at 8:00 AM. She was scheduled for 8:00.

AS: That's an important bit of information. They didn't make her wait unduly long. She could have known perhaps an hour earlier.

SY: But they checked earlier to find out about the blood, and they knew she wasn't going to go. Anyway I told the patient she wasn't going to surgery and she wept bitterly. She said, "It's cruel, it's cruel, I can't stand another day of this pain. They *must* do the surgery today; they *have* to do the surgery today." She said this in a high-pitched, screeching voice. I explained that I knew how she felt because of the pain and the buildup that had occurred (you know, holding it off and holding it off), but that they couldn't do the surgery because blood was not available. She kept saying, "I've *got* to have it done today. I've *got* to have it done today." Then she said, "I don't think that they are really going to do the surgery. They are just going to put it off and put it off, and they are really not going to do it." Then with great desperation, "They have got to have it done today." She just *wept* in *bitter, real despair*—anger and everything was all mixed up in it. There was nothing I could do, and she wept for at least a half an hour. I felt *terrible* for her, poor lady. I thought, "My God, she has really got a reason for despair and crying." I stood there throughout all of this, and I thought, "I feel like leaving but I can't leave." I was holding her hand while she was crying. After this was over, I went out into the hallway and said to the head nurse, "You know, Mrs. Abel is really upset about the surgery." She answered, "Well I thought this would happen," and she just shook her head. The other nurses whom I told just shook their heads and said, "It's terrible, it's terrible." But *nobody* came into the room. As a matter of fact, nobody has ever come into the room during the time that I have taken care of Mrs. Abel.

AS: Now you are catching their sympathy at the choices confronting the woman. Yet that doesn't mean that they are able to care better for her.

SY: It's interesting, too, that during these days it's one aide or another that is assigned to the patient. And she is the kind of patient that is complicated enough to require a registered nurse.

AS: How was the aide taking it that day?

SY: Something has to be done—is the feeling I get, what can she do about it? She's very happy when I go in and talk to the patient, and she won't come in when I am in there. She says, "Oh, you're busy with the patient." Any kind of excuse.

Throughout the morning Mrs. Abel would say, "They have *got* to do it; they *have* to do it today." I would be bathing her and all of a sudden she would come out with this. I would say I knew how she felt and then she would settle down, but then it would be reopened again.

AS: Nobody ever told her why they were not operating? And that when they schedule an operation for a given hour that if it isn't done you have to wait for the next day?

SY: No. Well she knew the blood was not available but apparently nobody had told her about this problem of the blood. I did tell her. She said: "What difference does it make, what difference does it make whether they have the blood or not. I am going to die anyway." There was nothing I could say. Just that the surgeons didn't want to risk the surgery without blood.

AS: Did you feel she understood what you were saying about the technicality of giving blood?

SY: She knew but she didn't want to be reasonable about it . . . I told her they were going to have some problems getting the blood, trying to prepare her for the fact that maybe the operation was going to be delayed more than just a day or so.

AS: In the last three weeks or so, how intensely rational she is by comparison with her previous months here. Although she is, as you say, being irrational here—"I want it, I want it, I want it" —still she is intensely rational in facing up to real issues.

SY: Anyway, her breakfast had become cold as a result of this episode, so I warmed it up for her. I might add that there has been a tremendous amount of hassling over cold breakfasts. The nurses' notes say, "Be with patient with her meals because she falls asleep." Many times I have gone by to see her at noon time and she was asleep over her meal. Nobody had awakened her so I'd wake her and chat while she was eating, and I'd run out to the icebox where she had a little box of special food and get things for her. She would say, "They know that I always want this thing from the icebox whenever I eat my lunch and dinner, but they *never* bring it."

AS: Did you ever see a dietician on the floor in all this time?

SY: No. Earlier when this cold meal hassle was going on, I had posed to her the possibility of cold cereal because even at best, the hospital's hot cereal is not hot. Her answer was that she didn't like cold cereal all the time. Then I asked the staff what kind of combinations could be made, and they said they just couldn't be bothered with all her little whims. Anyway, the thing that fascinated me was that after each cold meal hassle she would whimper and cry for about an hour. And I thought, golly it only takes about ten minutes at the most to warm this meal up, and it would save the staff putting up with all this whimpering and they never . . .

AS: But they would lose the battle.

SY: Yes. I thought, "My God, it is just a plain old power struggle, nothing else matters at this point any more, it is a power struggle"! The other thing that fascinated me as I stayed with her was that she ate a good breakfast despite her looking so terrible. In fact, all the mornings I had her, she always ate well and dwelt a great deal upon food dislikes and likes. At the time I was taking care of my aunt when she died of cancer, I was also astonished at how much she ate: she talked about wanting to die and at the same time there was this almost desperate eating, as if it was the thing that kept a person going. You know: "I want to die, but I want to live at the same time," and getting food was an important part of the process. Well, as I was watching Mrs. Abel, I thought of the strange form that wanting to live can take and wondered, too, if this eating met certain kinds of needs that the staff was not capable of supplying. Anyway, as I said earlier, throughout the four and one-half hours I was with her she wept, and I was *exhausted* at the end of the morning!

She behaved similarly to how she had behaved when I first began to take care of her: making demands one right after another, seeming to be afraid that I would leave her. I would have to reassure her all morning long that if I went out I would be right back. Actually she did this for the first two weeks that I took care of her. After that she didn't need constantly to make demands on me.

SA: Is this the day she offered you money to stay?

SY: Yes. I thought that probably because I hadn't been in to give her direct care for about two and a half weeks she had to put me through the paces—and that as she gets worse, she is going to fall back on her old coping patterns, only probably more so.

SA: You also told me that day that you didn't feel she was now capable of bathing herself but that the staff was making her continue to do this, although Mrs. Abel protested. I asked you what you thought of her condition—was she able to do this?—and you said no.

SY: No, she was very weak and her skin was incontinent. I thought I'd better watch her skin, so I bathed her. She said the nurses were insisting that she bathe herself and that she found this very difficult to do because her arms and legs were becoming so heavy and she was getting so weak. Also that the nurses were making her move, trying to make her move rapidly, and she couldn't do this because of the heaviness of the legs. During the bathing, the slightest amount of pressure would cause her to whimper. She reminded me of a whimpering, scared child, the kind that we see up in pediatrics.

SA: You also said Mrs. Abel was complaining that the staff was treating her like a child. You said that they were inconsistent. (This was the time that she fell again when trying to get out to the commode, and so the orders went up again that she was not to be left alone and the side rails had to be left up. The day staff were following through on this order but the evening staff wasn't.) So there was some vacillation and inconsistency, again with the legal aspects being hinted, with the possibility of a suit even at this late date. You also said that Mrs. Abel was complaining that the nurses were treating her like a child.

SY: At one point she said that she hoped that the hypophysectomy would not cause a hormonal imbalance and that it was easy to correct. "I don't want to be big and fat." It struck me: here she is one minute talking of wanting to die ("I want to have the surgery today") and yet saying, "Is it going to cause hormonal imbalance?" Then she said the surgery would cause her to die twice. I asked, "die twice?" She stated the surgery might help for a period, and she might not have pain, but eventually she would have to face again the fact of dying. So I said, "Yes, you mean you would have to face it again," trying to get her to discuss it further, but she didn't answer. At the end of the morning Mrs. Abel *begged* me to come back because she didn't think she could stand another day.

AS: It sounds like surgery represented not simply the release of pain but a release from having to face death, facing it over and over again each day.

SA: Yes, because later, on February 25, the change came; she accepted the fact that death was inevitable, imminent. But the days that we are talking about now are the 11th and 12th of February. So each day she had to face this during that period of time. And without very many people around. Almost everybody has pulled out. You were away on vacation from the campus during that period of time. I was away. The chaplain was in to see her a little, but she was pretty isolated during that period.

AS: In a teaching hospital, these are the kinds of timing accidents that do occur. This means that the most important person to her (meaning you, Shizu) had pulled out. She knew why you had pulled out, she wasn't blaming you, but she really had nobody there. Even if Shirley had still been on the case, she would also have been away. It also looks as though the chaplain was away because this was his opportunity to do things away from the hospital.

SA: So she really was pretty much alone, not because people had pulled out intentionally.

SY: On February 14, I went up to see the patient and the staff said, "The same as usual." Then when I asked June how Mrs. Abel

142

was doing, she said, "She is sleeping now," as if to say, "Don't go over to talk to her and wake her up." I went by the patient's room and she was sleeping soundly. I thought of calling to her but thought better of it, because if I awakened her she would disturb the staff, and they would never forgive me. The night nurse's notation earlier that morning was: "Patient said, 'Please don't leave, I will die if you leave me.'" As I read it I thought how sad that everybody is rejecting Mrs. Abel, and she is facing death all alone without any comfort and without any type of understanding. The assistant head nurse, Elaine, stated that surgery was rescheduled for the following Tuesday, and I said, "Are they really going to do the surgery; it seems kind of late." Her response was, "Isn't it sad, isn't it terrible." And she shook her head. When I asked how long she thought the patient was going to live, she didn't know. She had predicted the patient would die about Christmas time and was surprised how long the patient lived. "Aren't you shocked to see her change from day to day. You know, I've been off for two days and she has sunk so fast."

On the 17th she looked terrible. A graduate nurse was taking care of her. I helped take care of her. The patient stated, "I hope the surgery works. I hope it works." Then Dr. Colp came in and examined the patient's heart and lungs very carefully and asked, "Are there any new complaints you have?" He examined the chest so carefully I thought he must be really concerned about her respiratory state. Then he impressed on the patient that the surgery might help, but then it might not, and that he didn't know the actual statistics but there was not 100% relief from pain. He asked if the neurologist had answered all the questions she might have. He remarked that she should try to see the nuerosurgeon this morning so that her questions would get adequate answers. "I want you to be sure that this is what you want and have all your questions answered, because the neurosurgeons would be very upset if you changed your mind at the last minute." I was thinking, "My God, she should care less about how the neurosurgeons felt"! Also, "My God, he's asking her to be responsible"! During all of this she was listening very thoughtfully. Then she asked the doctor if the swelling in the legs would go down after the surgery. The physician answered that he didn't know.

AS: Had she, by the way, ever commented to you about the swelling and the breaking of the skin in her leg?

SY: Yes, she was very disturbed about it. She knew things just were not working.

AS: What did the doctor answer when she asked?

143

SY: He didn't know what it was—but they could replace the hormones.

As he left the room, he re-emphasized again that she should be sure that her question about the neurosurgery be clarified with the neurosurgeon. Then when he left the room, he said to me, "*God* I hate coming up here, it's *so* depressing." He expressed a great deal of concern about Mrs. Abel's physical condition, wondering if she would be able to tolerate this surgery. He said, "I just don't know whether the surgeons will do the surgery in her condition." He stopped the head nurse and asked that the neurosurgeons be called to come and see the patient this morning because he wanted the neurosurgeons to be sure to see her physical state and also to answer any questions that Mrs. Abel might have. He said that he was sorry that the surgery had been delayed for so long; it might have been a different matter had it been done at the time it was originally proposed.

AS: Yet he cannot draw back and say "no surgery" at this moment.

SY: So I asked, "What's going to happen if the surgeons decide to cancel the surgery because of her poor physical state?" And I described the tremendous anxiety shown by the patient in the last episode. "Gee, I don't know, I don't know." The head nurse was listening to the conversation, and she shook her head in great dismay.

AS: Actually he could have said "no," but he didn't. Have you any idea why not?

SA: He felt this was the only thing that was left. They were not able to stop her pain. They had done everything else possible. She had been on all the hormone drugs that were possible—and *this* was the last resort.

SY: He wanted to be sure that the patient understood that the relief of pain was not positive after the surgery, and he felt perhaps that he should make a notation on the chart that the patient had been informed of this. "You know, she has a history of suing." Later I checked on the chart; he had not made a notation about this. He felt that the patient's life would now be only a matter of days.

I asked him how long he expected the patient to live when originally admitted in October. Perhaps five or six months. Somewhere around there. But he added that he had *never* been able to predict the survival time of his patients. Although he did say that the patients always seemed to die earlier than he predicted.

SA: So he is predicting two or three days now?

SY: As he left the unit he volunteered, "God I *hate* coming up on this unit, it is so depressing." That was the last comment I heard from him before the surgery. I went back to the patient's room and again she said she hoped that the surgery would work because she just simply could not tolerate the pain anymore. Then in the next breath, she hoped to die.

I told her that I would be in to take care of her and would be in the surgery with her, and she said, "Thank God." In other words, somebody was going to be with her that cared about her. I did consider staying with her that evening, but I had a dinner engagement. I wanted to be with her. Yet I had a real sense of guilt as I left her because I was concerned about the clipping of her hair and all the other things that would be involved if they decided to do the surgery. I still wasn't sure whether the neurosurgeons were going to do the surgery or not. I believed more than likely they would not because of her physical state and certainly from what Dr. Colp had said.

That night I had people over to dinner and I didn't think about her. I conked out at the ungodly hour of about 2:00 AM. Before I did, I asked my house guest to wake me up because I *had* to go on duty tomorrow morning on time.

The social worker stated that she felt Mrs. Abel really wanted the surgery and had asked her if the medical staff would continue to keep her alive with intravenous feedings after she became comatose—she hoped they would not.

AS: Mrs. Abel never said anything like that to you?

SY: No. The social worker added that in the earlier encounters, the patient would ask her to do things, and the social worker explained to her that she was very happy to do these things, but she really wanted to spend the time talking to her about other matters. How she realized that there was little she could do in terms of comforting the patient because the nursing staff was incapable of being with Mrs. Abel and that these little acts were comforting to her. She said, "You know, it's sad the power struggle that goes on between Mrs. Abel and the staff." About Mrs. Abel's question about being comatose, she answered that she was not in the medical field and could not answer the question.

AS: Shirley I want to ask you whether in your last interview with Dr. Colp he indicated, in any way, that at the end he also was responsible for having caused the death of the patient through an error of judgment (having to do with chest fluid, and so on, as described by the chief neurosurgeon)?

SA: He did not directly state this. He discussed the differences of prognosis which went into the neurosurgeons' decision to do surgery and how their decision was predicated upon the information that *he* gave them. They made the final decision to do this. He was quite aware of his error of judgment which, although not directly stated, was indirectly implied by, "Maybe I should have checked on the [floors]," and "Maybe I should have done a potassium, but I thought thus and so on . . . before surgery, that potassium was . . . ."

AS: "Maybe I should have checked on . . . ." is a different thing than what the head neurosurgeon told you, which was that he was really responsible because *that* was what really did it. In other words, does Dr. Colp know that *that* was what really *did* it?

SA: He said that she died . . . she stopped breathing, she had a cardiac arrest.

SY: He said there were multiple causes, although following the surgery he realized that there was some brain stem dysfunction because of the fact that the patient's eyes, the pupils, were not reacting.

AS: We're going to record now what has been happening in the last week or so since Mrs. Abel's death; for instance, I had asked Shirley if she wouldn't check out how the decision was made to put this woman onto the operating table.

SA: I'll combine Dr. Wallace's and Dr. Colp's account. Dr. Wallace is the chief resident for the Neurosurgery Department, and I was finally able to get hold of him. I asked whether he could tell me something about Mrs. Abel. "Well, she was a hopeless case," meaning that she was a great bother to the girls on the floor. He said that the hypophysectomy was done for regression of her tumor, but that it is very rarely done for pain. This is the story I get from most of the surgeons—there is real discrepancy about whether pain relief is actually a primary reason for doing this surgery. There is one piece of literature re pain, and I had worked with one patient who was in the same kind of pain that I had cared for post-hypophysectomy, so I was baiting him with information from these sources. He said it was partially done for pain, but it was also done for tumor regression. He went on, "She really doesn't have pain," and I said, "Oh." He said, "If you ever listen to her, she doesn't complain of pain, she complains of tightness in her chest, and she just can't cope with it." He said, "Her chest and her arms look horrible." I don't know if he knew I had actually seen the patient. Then he went on to say, "I'm a junior man in a large overall group, and I don't make the decisions but follow them." When I pushed him a little further, he meant by this that a private consultant had made the choice of surgery. Dr. Wallace would have preferred a lobotomy, but Dr. Stanton made the decision for the hypophysectomy.

When I saw Dr. Stanton—he made the final decision about the kind of surgery—to find out why he had selected the hypophysectomy, I found out that he had designed the operation originally. He's the first to have done a hypophysectomy. I just assumed from my own experience that it was the doctor I worked with in New York, Dr. Bray. Dr. Stanton feels that Dr. Bray might have done more hypophysectomies, but he originated it and has done the basic research for the hypophysectomy. I started asking him about . . .

AS: You started to say first that you discovered that he had invented it and how odd that nobody around here knew it.

SA: Yes. Everytime I talked to any of the physicians who were in on the case I was getting this two-fold thing: "Yes, it is done for pain," or "No, it isn't done for pain," and "This surgery is always used for secondary to relief regression of tumor." Shizu also was getting this from all the doctors. When now I asked Dr. Stanton why this was done, he said, "Well, it's done for pain, and you might possibly get some regression of tumor." I said, "Is there any physiological reason for wanting to relieve pain?" He said, "No, I can't give that to you, it isn't scientifically proven yet and what little there is it would take a volume to do this." So I asked why the lobotomy was not done (you know, it was under consideration). He said there really isn't any scientific research done of the effects of lobotomy, and if there was someone here who was qualified to do a lobotomy I suppose we might have considered letting him do it for research purposes, if no questions would have been asked. Everybody gave me this same information in terms of the hypophysectomy: there's no research done, no statistical data coming out about the effects of this.

AS: But they all, including the doctors, did buy the idea that a lobotomy will reduce pain?

SA: Yes, this is why the lobotomy is done, it produces euphoria and so forth. But Dr. Stanton was saying there's no scientific research that validates that, and the other physicians are saying, "There's no scientific research that validates the hypophysectomy."

AS: Who was actually considering doing this lobotomy?

SA: Dr. Colp, at Dr. Tree's suggestion, asked for a consultation for a lobotomy to be done. Dr. Wallace wanted to do a lobotomy. Dr. Stanton, when this came up for his review, said to do the hypophysectomy instead.

AS: Did he give those reasons to Dr. Wallace, do you know?

SA: I doubt it from what Dr. Wallace said. I asked Dr. Wallace, "Why is Dr. Stanton doing this?" He said, "For the same reason that you just said—cut down on pain and secondarily for the regression of the tumor." When I asked him if it were his private patient what would he have done, he said, "I would have done a lobotomy, but Dr. Stanton is my chief, he's my consult, and his word . . ." Anyway, Dr. Stanton decided that they would do the hypophysectomy. Dr. Wallace said, "It was an error to do surgery. It was an error in judgment of Mrs. Abel's capacity to tolerate it. If the physician, the internist—meaning Dr. Colp—and the radiologist had indicated to us the amount of fluid in her chest cavity, and the degree of which her reserve was limited, her lung capacity, we would not have done surgery." He felt that her death was due to the fact that she was a poor surgical risk, but they had not known it, it didn't show up in their X-rays, or the internist and radiologist had not indicated it—one of the two.

AS: Which did he think it was—did he give any indication?

SA: He said either/or. Dr. Colp knew there was fluid in the chest. In fact, he said, "Maybe we should have withdrawn some of the fluid before we did surgery, but I don't think it would have made any difference." He was evaluating in his mind when I talked with him the last time.

SY: He knew there was fluid because he examined the patient's chest very carefully the day before she went to surgery. I thought, "Aha, he worried about this," and I discussed it with him afterwards.

AS: So he made a calculated judgment on this?

SA: He felt it was not going to affect her ability to tolerate surgery.

SY: Dr. Wallace had seen the patient a week prior. The PM nurse saw Dr. Wallace and asked about the surgical risk involved, and he said that he felt that the patient would pull through fine.

AS: On the basis of his own examination or on the basis of conversations with . . . ?

SA: When we checked this out—as to who said what to each other about the prognosis—there must have been confused communication between the two of them, or very little, if any, and strictly on the charts.

AS: What do we know about the radiologist's report?

SY: They were concerned with the bone metastases. They did calcium studies, and they did . . .

SA: Did they do chest X-rays prior to surgery? Dr. Colp didn't mention a word.

SY: I don't know. They did do an EKG on her.

SA: Yes, and because the neurologist had not written orders for the routine pre-op exams, Dr. Colp picked it up and did, but he didn't mention having a chest X-ray. But that's not necessarily routine, pre-operatively.

AS: The only point I'm getting at here is establishing the *kind* of error that was made.

SA: Dr. Stanton meant that it was not simply lack of communication, but of what information they had to evaluate her real surgical risk as a candidate.

SA: Dr. Wallace said, "You know that she's a terrible surgical risk. Then how do you go about deciding whether you do surgery or not? She's never going to get any better, and therefore you base on that your assessment on whether to do surgery or not." And he said he had judged she had a fair longevity. At the moment he didn't think her lesions were threatening. This is the impression he got from Dr. Colp when originally he talked to him about the consultation—that probably she had one to six months' prognosis and that the lesions then were still superficial to the skin. They were not spread to the vital organs yet. When I asked him, "Well, were you relieved at her death?" he said, "Oh, no, we were disappointed—although she's a CA patient so it's not quite the disappointment that we might have if she were another kind of patient. But we were still disappointed because we wouldn't have done the surgery if we didn't think we could help her." The two phrases that came through to me were that he said she was "a terrible risk" and it was "a disappointment."

SY: The social worker talked to him two weeks prior to the surgery. Dr. Wallace had said at that time that the patient was asking us to kill her. And also that the operation is not being done to stop pain but for this tightness. It was not pain but tightness—Dr. Colp had told us and the patient also—so the following day I questioned the patient rather closely to find out how she felt about it. She reassured me over and over again that it was *real* pain. Also, in reference to lobotomy, she said that it was done to relieve anxiety.

AS: Did she see Wallace before the operation?

SY: Yes, she went into great detail about what the surgeons had told her, particularly of the lobotomy.

SA: I went to Dr. Colp to find out what was actually going on because we had gotten the impression from Dr. Colp that by the time they got around to doing surgery he didn't think Mrs. Abel's condition was as good as when he first asked for a consult with Dr. Wallace. So I asked him to describe her condition during her last few weeks while they were making the decision of surgery. He started talking about the four or five weeks prior to the actual surgical procedure: he had asked for consults (it was on the 1st of January) for a possible lobotomy. He did this because Dr. Tree who had been doing the research suggested that the only thing that might help Mrs. Abel was a lobotomy. Dr. Colp followed up on Dr. Tree's suggestion and had a neuro consult. In the beginning he had not thought of a hypophysectomy because the experience here in again that if the patient hadn't obtained relief for regression of tumor on hormonal therapy, then a hypophysectomy didn't help either. So since she had not had regression of tumor, he hadn't even considered a hypophysectomy. However, he also indicated that pain relief was discussed in one piece of literature. He and I talked about it back in September when discussing Mrs. Abel and the kinds of surgical procedures that were available. I had asked him if they ever did do hypophysectomies here, and he gave me essentially the same information then and even brought up the article I was familiar with. He mentioned again the other day that there was literature about the procedures being useful for pain relief. He said that when they first started considering it, the neurosurgeons hadn't communicated too often with him. Two or three weeks after he asked for the consult he suddenly discovered that they were planning a lobotomy, but were going to use some special stereotaxic equipment which was unavailable at the time because it needed to be repaired. At this time also Dr. Colp was out of town for almost a week at a conference. So he said communications had been really infrequent, most of it written on the chart, what little there was, and that occasionally he called the neurosurgeons or they would call him about it. So finally about a week prior to surgery when the hypophysectomy was decided on, they apparently notified him or put it on the chart that hypophysectomy was the operation decided upon. He cleared it with Dr. Saite who is the head of the Breast Tumor Research Clinic and who is Dr. Colp's chief. Dr. Saite said—although Dr. Colp didn't feel he would normally have suggested this procedure —that in this particular case they would try anything. Then surgery was scheduled almost a week before it was actually done. And when they started to obtain blood, they found that Mrs. Abel had blood incompatabilities; they were running into antigen antibody reactions on the blood and had to postpone surgery again. On the Friday prior to surgery, Dr. Colp realized that they had not ordered some of the routine procedural lab requirements. He checked to see if the neurosurgeons were going to order hemoglobin. The neurosurgeons told him to go ahead and order it, so he ordered the routine kind of lab procedures that would be required for surgery. The only procedure he didn't order was one for potassium, which is not necessarily routine, I don't think. He felt that maybe she might have been low in potassium, but the probabilities were she was not, because he had been giving massive doses of potassium. The only other thing we might have done, in retrospect, he said, was "we might have tapped the chest for fluid in the chest." "I don't really think that would have made any difference."

AS: What's the meaning of the neurosurgeons not having ordered the routine tests?

SA: By and large, they were waiting for Dr. Colp to do all the ordering. She was never transferred to the neurosurgery service. Also, Dr. Colp again mentioned that during the last two weeks he had cut narcotics, and she was now down from 24 mg of morphine to 12 mg and received no other sedatives. Her tolerance was then about four to five times greater than the average person.

SY: I might add that the phenobarbital and sparine which had been given between each narcotic injection was now discontinued.

SA: She was not then complaining about pain, therefore Dr. Colp felt that 95% of her pain had been due to anxiety. Then he described another patient who in the last few weeks of her life, like Mrs. Abel, developed massive lesions at her throat, but didn't complain of pain until the last few days of her life. Mrs. Abel is going the other way, she had complained of massive pain, but now right at the end she isn't. "Another thing I noticed about these patients is that none of them die comatose. They are all alert." He said that the nurse will go in and just find them dead, although they had just been talking a little while before. "There's nothing routine about the way these people die, so you never know what to expect. This is why I don't give a definite prognosis, and then it's always in terms of from one to six months, from one to two years. Finally with Mrs. Abel I probably told the neurosurgeons one to six months, particularly when I first asked for a consult. If they had asked me for it the days of surgery, it would probably have been one day to three months, but even then I could have said six months."

AS: What were the nurses anticipating just before the operation about the length of time Mrs. Abel had to live?

SY: There were mixed responses. Elaine felt that the patient was going to die around Christmas time and was surprised that the patient hung on as long as she did. Two or three days before the operation, she wasn't sure that . . . all she did was shake her head when I asked. She couldn't predict what was going to happen. Mrs. Abel had lived so much longer than . . . The others kind of shook their heads, not being sure because she had dragged on longer, but they knew her death was pretty close. And I predicted, I predicted probably around two weeks at the most.

SA: They told me the same thing.

SA: Anyway Dr. Colp felt that these people can look very awake and be dead the next minute, or they can hang on and drag and drag. At this time the staff and he weren't even talking to each other. He wasn't on the floor at all, there was no communication.

SY: It is interesting that when neurosurgery was being posed, and the doctor went on vacation and came back, there was a great big sign on the chart saying the neurosurgeons can do whatever they want.

SA: This was probably after Dr. Colp talked to Dr. Saite. He was not really expecting Mrs. Abel to die on the table, and he still felt this was the proper procedure to do. Mrs. Abel was uncomfortable for one thing and there wasn't any other alternative to offer for pain relief. "The length of life is not so important," he said, "but rather the productivity and the comfortableness of the person and whether they are able to be productive. Therefore, the length of life is not necessarily important." He said, "Although I felt there was some risk involved, the procedure might help, but what did we have to lose."

And she might get regression of her disease, and she might get pains, so she wouldn't improve otherwise. There was no other possibility of relief. This was when (Elaine told me) he was cutting medications because her pain was decreasing. He did everything else to keep her comfortable. This was the last resort to keep her comfortable—and no one would complain. He emphasized this. And he seemed less emotionally involved when talking in a more objective way about the various processes of the disease. He spent a whole hour on it, right through his lunch hour. He had just finished one conference and had another appointment with someone else, but he spent the whole hour with me. He said she had inflammatory carcinoma which is about 2% of all the CA's. But it's one of the most rapid growing of cancers. This is the one CA you do not do surgery for. The biopsy was done simply to make the diagnosis. There was absolutely nothing that could be done for her when she originally went to her doctor. Remember Mrs. Abel complaining that if the original doctor she had seen had done something about it perhaps she would have lived, or wouldn't have been in such pain? There was *nothing* that could be done. This was a terminal CA and there was nothing you could do for it.

AS: Did he tell the patient?

SA: He said, "I told her that, but she never was able to accept it, she always complained that if only someone had done something earlier."

AS: So he was justifying what he'd done, although very battered about the whole experience.

SA: That's right . . . . I also interviewed—on the telphone— the scrub nurse from the operating room. She's the lady whom Shizu described earlier as having picked up the patient for surgery. This nurse's description was, "Poor woman, it would have been a blessing if she could have been 'taken' on the table, because she was in such agony when I went to get her." She repeated this innumerable times. She said very little about the procedure, but it was done in order to make her more comfortable. I asked her if this was actually said in the operating room. "No, but this is something we know, we don't do very many of them, but it is common knowledge that this is the purpose it is done for." There was some discussion that with the procedure Mrs. Abel might have actually lived for another two years. "Our response was 'heaven forbid,' she's already suffered too much" and that Mrs. Abel just couldn't endure this longer; "she was in absolute agony. I don't know how she could tolerate it."

SA: From her first contact with Mrs. Abel that morning when she went after her to bring her to surgery. She also described the nurses on the floor as not being too cooperative. "The poor woman was calling for a nurse when I went after her. There was an aide standing outside of the room and just standing in the hallway talking, and I couldn't even get her to help me get Mrs. Abel on the guerney. Finally, she was in such excrutiating pain that I just said to one of them, 'can't you give us a hand,' or something or other on that order." Then she added, "Before Mrs. Abel went to sleep, she said, 'I don't care if I die on the table.'" She was amazed that with the excrutiating pain this woman had something had not been done earlier for her. Why wasn't the operation done earlier? Why was she being kept in the hospital? "I looked at the chart and realized she was in since November. How can she be in the hospital this long without anybody doing anything for her?" Taking up the

153

research bed at forty dollars a day—and it had to be a private room because if there was another patient in the room Mrs. Abel would decrease his morale. "If it was a comatose patient in the room, then it would decrease Mrs. Abel's morale. So it would have to be a private room." She didn't understand: this was wasted bed space.

Finally she told me more about the surgery. There had been a lot of people in the room as this is a rather unique procedure, not done very often. Everybody was in the room to see the operation. Everybody regarded this as a pathetic case. She went on to describe Mrs. Abel's condition to me, and the discussion that occurred in the operating room about the massive spreading. She had never seen spreading like this. She had never seen one that had spread so massively without something being done. "I've been in the OR long enough, and I've seen a lot of metastatic CA." She said, Dr. Wallace asked his assistant to look at the opposite breast and to realize how hard and firm it was and that the metastases had moved that far over."

This nurse then said to me: "The patient will be so helpless and will have to be taken care of and probably will still be in pain because of the extensiveness of the disease in spite of the surgery." (She didn't know Mrs. Abel was dead, and I had not told her. We had been talking twenty to thirty minutes.) I said, "Eileen, can you tell me what you thought of Mrs. Abel's condition just prior to surgery in terms of operative risk?" She said, "I really couldn't say." She was thinking, and I asked, "Well, you know, you go after a lot of surgical patients and you usually make some kind of judgment about whether you think they're going to die on the table, or do they look comatose, or do they look in pretty bad shape when going into OR?" She said, "Oh, not in such good shape, but can't make a judgment." I never could get her to make a judgment on what *she* thought. In spite of the fact that she is my friend, and that having been an OR nurse myself, you do make these decisions. I have a hunch she thought the patient never should have gone on the table. This is just a hunch. She wanted the patient to die on the table. The patient did not die, but it's still a hunch that she thought the patient was a pretty bad surgical risk.

She also said that the patient was not capable of making a rational decision at this point; she was in so much misery and pain that she was beyond thinking whether or not the procedure should be done, but just wanted anything done that would offer her relief. So I asked, "Well, how about the neurosurgeons? Did they seem to want to do the surgery?" Although nothing was said specifically in the OR, Eileen got the impression that they were a little bit reluctant

154

and that pressure was coming from the patient's physician. (She didn't know who Dr. Colp was.) One of the nurses in passing said that this patient really makes you believe in euthanasia for "religious or moral reasons. No one can take the responsibility for killing someone; but if there was an accident or something, it would only be for the best." Eileen again repeated, "It would have been a real blessing if she could have gone on the table." She's been a surgical nurse for five or six years. The nurse who made the comment about euthanasia was the chief of the neurosurgical room. I decided then to say, "You know, Mrs. Abel died the night following surgery." There was just silence at the other end of the phone . . . She said, "I'm glad to hear that." The death came as a complete surprise to her. There had been no follow-up to see what happened to this patient at all. It had not been discussed in the operating rooms because I asked if there had been any discussion at all. It had *not* been discussed at all.

AS: I have the impression also that ordinarily there is little flowback from ICU to surgery.

SA: If there is a great deal of interest by the nurse—medical interest and concern—then she will find out. This is a large hospital, too, so you rarely get word back otherwise . . . . Eileen went on to ask, "Couldn't she have been placed in a rest home before? Why did she take up the hospital bed?" She actually said they misused the hospital. She didn't realize either that previous surgery hadn't been done. This is the reason I pushed Dr. Colp and cleared up the question for my own satisfaction—because she felt there had been some politics, that the patient had been kept because somebody goofed.

SY: I talked to this nurse before she scrubbed in for surgery. She was going on and on, very angry, at what she had to go through to get the patient onto the stretcher, and nobody helping her—and on and on and on.

AS: One thing is now apparent. The decision to operate was made by Dr. Colp. But the decision to use this particular kind of procedure was made by Dr. Stanton. And the man who actually did the operating was asked to use this procedure and was familiar with it but would rather have used another procedure—namely, the lobotomy.

SA: Dr. Wallace had never done a hypophysectomy before. He's the chief resident of neurosurgery. They don't do these very often. He ran into trouble and had to have Dr. Stanton in. They simply don't do that many hypophysectomies and they're tricky. Dr. Stanton is quite familiar with hypophysectomy.

SY: I talked to Helen and she said that during the operation the ward went on per usual. They were taking care of their assigned patients, and she was concerned mostly about another patient that had been sent up to surgery. He was a young fellow. Right after she got home from duty she thought of calling the floor to find out what had happened, but her roommate talked her out of it. She was going to call specifically about this young patient, not Mrs. Abel. No one on the ward called the OR to find out what was going on with Mrs. Abel.

AS: *The whole day.*

SY: The whole day! They found out that Mrs. Abel died the following morning when Dr. Wallace happened to get off the elevator, but nobody asked. I would say this is unusual—well, I don't know.

SA: Not unless the family is there. Families are usually there checking. Or again for a particular interest or reason.

AS: Such as the highly valued patient. Otherwise they will not check. Ordinarily the patient will go to the ICU and the cancer ward will eventually find out what happened. In fact, the patient might never return to their floor.

SY: Helen said a couple of patients asked about Mrs. Abel because they heard her being wheeled out. They knew her. Helen said that after three days on the ward, the patients knew about Mrs. Abel and asked about her, because she generally cried during the night, and this is how they knew her. The staff explained that Mrs. Abel was going up to surgery and would be transferred to another unit, and no patient asked any questions after that.

Then Helen went on: she was quite critical about how Dr. Colp handled the situation. He told the nurses one thing and told the patient another.

Then she went on in detail about how the patient manipulated everybody and even manipulated other patient's visitors and other patients, and the battle over a specific chair that faced the big window, and how another patient who used to give in to Mrs. Abel once put her foot down.

Then she said she was leaving in July. She had applied for a job at the VA Hospital. I asked how long she had stayed. About a year and a half. I said she had been here a long time. "I must be nuts for remaining so long on this unit." She's the same nurse who, about November when all these deaths were taking place and Mrs. Abel continued to stay, said that she was really beginning to realize the ward was a very depressing place, and she had been fighting with herself, not going into the patient's room as often as she used to when she first came on the job.

SA: I talked to Helen's roommate yesterday, a classmate of mine, and asked her if she noticed anything. Does Helen seem the same, anxious, happier? She indicated it's hard to evaluate because Helen had been in a car accident the last week. But she knew exactly what I meant, I was thinking in terms of her work. She knew Helen was certainly relieved about Mrs. Abel. This was discussed at home, and her roommate knew exactly what I was talking about, even the kind of procedure done. *She* expressed an opinion that surgery never should have been done.

SY: The two aides confirmed this. They said they are very busy with other patients and they didn't think about Mrs. Abel. Both said she was one of the most difficult patients they had ever taken care of, and they felt badly for her when she was wheeled off to surgery. "No matter how annoying or irritating a person might be, you just can't help but feel something toward the patient." The patient talked a lot about dying and had said she wanted to die. But the aide didn't feel the patient had really accepted death because she kept talking about the time she would go home after the surgery. Then one aide said that she didn't mind taking care of the patient so much if she hadn't of had the other patients to take care. The other aide said she was being assigned more frequently to Mrs. Abel, where previously the assignment was more evenly divided. She was a little irritated (of course, I baited her into it). Actually I did notice whenever I went to see the patient that usually the aide was bathing the patient, during the last month. "Although Mrs. Abel was irritating and very exacting about her appearance and how things were done, I do give her credit for being concerned about her appearance." Some other patients in the terminal state just let themselves go.

AS: These are the only nice things we're hearing about Mrs. Abel—and from the aides.

SA: That's true right from the start.

SY: The social worker talked to the husband on the floor last week. She said that he seemed amazingly calm and said the funeral had taken place the day before, and since he was in such an agitated state the social worker wanted to be sure that he had somebody to go to if he needed help. He said he had been going to his own private physician and was taking tranquilizers. The RN on the evening shift said that Mr. Abel was quite agitated and upset the night before surgery. He made the statement then that he didn't think he would ever see his wife again. He cried, and she felt terrible for the husband.

AS: Did she say what she did?

SY: She just listened to him. The social worker went on to say that early in January plans were made for the patient to be discharged. Three or four weeks following, Dr. Colp would call her about two times a week asking if plans had been confirmed for the discharge. She would keep telling him that plans had been made, but each time he would say, "Well, we're extending it for pain study." She kept thinking that she could get through to the patient until about three weeks prior to surgery. Then she decided that whatever she did was not going to make any difference, so all she could do was to comfort the patient by doing little things, such as fluffing her pillows, getting little things for her, and meeting small little requests that the patient had made to her. Because the social worker also realized that the nurses could not tolerate being with the patient for any length of time, and if this was comforting to the patient, she would do it.

SA: This is what the chaplain did.

AS: Both played somewhat the same role. Did he fluff her pillows?

SA: Yes, and straightened her position because she was uncomfortable.

SY: The social worker said the patient was indecisive about the hypophysectomy and had pressed her for an opinion—although not for the pain release as much as for the lobotomy. She felt that the patient saw the hypaphysectomy as a kind of "counter-irritant" to forget about pain. The social worker said she had never seen such a sick situation in all her life and hoped that she would never run into a situation like this again, but she had learned a great deal. She felt she could handle practically *anything* that came up now.

AS: What does she mean, she "learned"?

SY: Of how communications can get so garbled, the kinds of things that went on in terms of the dying patient.

AS: That's an instance of the mythology that things would be better if only communications could be better!

SY: And June said, "It's a real relief to have Mrs. Abel off, we can smile again." She thought the hypophysectomy was a crazy answer to the patient's problem, although she did not have another answer to it. She thought it was a senseless procedure.

SA: She must have thought the patient terminal then almost immediately, so that it was senseless to do it at this point—and also the patient was now more comfortable.

SY: Also, she said that Mrs. Abel was the most difficult patient she ever had. June never saw such a selfish person in all her life, and this was one patient she never could get through to and got no kind of positive response from. You don't expect patients to thank you all the time or appreciate everything, but some kind of interaction has to take place. She never got *anything* from this patient, who not once even said "thank you." Well, she did say thank you for little things but did not really mean it. I said, "Come to think of it, I never was thanked either," but I guess I wasn't looking for thanks.

Then she began to ask me questions: how did I make plans to go to school, who do I go to, and so on. She felt she learned quite a bit from the patient, awful as she was.

June was the one who said she thought it was a good thing that I had washed Mrs. Abel's hair, that it was the only thing the patient had left.

AS: June has shown a certain sensitivity all through even though she isn't able to maintain physical contact with the woman.

SY: The PM nurses said that two weeks prior to her death, Mrs. Abel became quieter, less agitated, although also getting more lethargic. She was amazingly quiet the night before the surgery. She also became docile after the head was shaved. The description I got was kind of eerily docile behavior. The PM nurses felt Mrs. Abel was looking upon the surgery as something that was finally being done for her and was looking forward to it.

SA: Don't you think they were rather surprised? This is the impression I got from you last night. This patient always complaining and all of a sudden she isn't complaining anymore. she was docile so she didn't fit their expectations.

AS: The surprise comes through very well as a kind of astonishment.

SA: Yes, it's amazing that they picked it up—because when a patient is a constant complainer, and although she may not complain *that* day, you still feel that she complained all the time. They picked it up that she was different.

SY: The husband used to visit Mrs. Abel in the evening, so the evening shift saw him most frequently. The staff said the husband was agitated three-quarters of the time, an agitation partly induced by the patient because she ordered him around and treated him pretty shabbily. One PM nurse said, "It's kind of a relief not to have the patient around but after you've had a patient as long as we've had, no matter how annoying and irritating a person might be, when they're gone all of a sudden you miss them."

I talked also to the visiting volunteer who began to see the patient around early November, at the request of the chaplain. She would come about one or one and a half hours every Thursday afternoon and would do little things for the patient like cutting her nails, rubbing her back, shampooing her hair, and meeting any kind of request that Mrs. Abel made. She said Mrs. Abel always cried a great deal just before she left. She realized what the patient was doing—wanted her to stay, and that's why the tears. She felt very, very sorry for the patient. "You could look at her and you knew that she had a lot of pain." She always had a good feeling after she'd been with the patient, that she had done something for this woman. She wasn't so sure if she would feel the same way about the patient if she had to take care of her for a long period of time. I asked if Mrs. Abel made critical statements about the nurses, and she hedged about it for a while. Then I began to describe the patient further, and then she remarked that if she were ever in a condition like Mrs. Abel, she would never die in a hospital. She cited instances of how difficult it was to get a nurse, and how long Mrs. Abel had to wait to get a pain pill, and that if she were in Mrs. Abel's shoes she would like to have people who were more personally interested. "I suppose though if you're around critically ill patients, and patients who are dying, for a long time, the nurse can't help but get a little hardened.

The volunteer is a very outgoing person, I guess in her late forties or early fifties. She reminded me of an adult girl scout. Middle-class, I would say. She had been doing this kind of work for the past four or five years.

AS: Did you know there was a volunteer with Mrs. Abel until recently?

SY: No. We were both surprised. We sat down and said, "Oh, you're the one that sees the patient two mornings a week." We ran into each other only three weeks prior to the death.

AS: How do you account for this lack of awareness?

SY: I don't know.

SA: The girls never mentioned her. I heard about her in December from the chaplain, and I never thought about it again be-

160

cause he never mentioned her, and I was never on the floor when she was there.

SY: She said she enjoyed doing things for the patients because she seemed to derive comfort from it. She realized the nurses were all so busy that they couldn't be doing all these things. Mrs. Abel cried a great deal and said that she wanted to die. She didn't blame the patient for feeling this way. She found it curious though that, at the same time, the patient asked her several times for her address, saying, "I want to write to you when I get out of the hospital."

AS: Shizu, I want to ask you about yourself now. What have the intervening days since Mrs. Abel's death been like for you?

SY: Relief that she's finally gone. I still have stomach disturbances so I guess I'm still in an uproar about it. It's made me realize more and more—although I got a glimmer of it—that it is not *enough* that the nurse understand herself better. You have to look around the patient to really know what's going on with the dying patient. There are certain things the nurse cannot do because of the other things going on around the patient which limit what she can do. It has made me realize that if I had *really* understood this better, I would probably not have had my gut in *quite* the uproar that I did at the time. On the other hand, it really taught me a great deal in terms of the cliche terms like body image, the relationship of pain to body image, and all those things. The cliches became very meaningful.

AS: Do you feel depressed now?

SY: No.

AS: What about the conversations we've been having? Have they had any effect?

SY: Yes, I think they have a cathartic value (in two ways)!

SA: I picked up a sense of depression in you, Shizu, last night when we talked. One area was when telling about the post-mortem conference.

SY: Chaplain Brinkley felt that there was a need for post-mortem conference with the nursing staff up there because he felt the staff was quite guilty about its feelings. I got the idea he wanted me roped into this thing, but I just didn't feel I could handle the situation. Then he made the statement that he felt that I was projecting the nurse's lack of readiness to do this.

AS: You say you couldn't handle the situation, meaning what?

161

SY: There were many periods while taking care of the patient when I really felt quite critical of the nursing staff. I thought that had they handled the situation differently, there wouldn't have been near the amount of whining and crying by the patient; and it would not help the purpose if I had to bring out some of these deep feelings. It wouldn't be good for the staff.

AS: It's interesting the chaplain believes that the staff members feel guilty and that somehow things would be better if they would talk a little. Do you agree?

SY: I'm not sure—if they just bring it out and don't do anything about it . . . . I was thinking it was too bad she didn't go home, so the staff could "work out" their feelings.

SA: In fact, at the time you were hoping she would. Chaplain Brinkley commented about the nurses in December. He felt they couldn't handle her because of guilt feelings, and spoke then of a conference, but decided to wait for a better time when they could look at it—as they were *so* involved. He was critical of the nurses because of their guilt and their inability to get over it. Dr. Colp was then talking at great length to me almost out of a need to talk.

SY: Now is the first time, in three weeks really, that the staff has been able to talk about Mrs. Abel to me. Prior to then, "Do what you like, don't bother me with this."

SA: Their immediate response was sudden relief and then talking, and then there had been two or three days of a guilt, depression, kind of feeling. Now a little more than a week later people are now beginning to talk at great length. There was a lull when they were working through their own feelings.

SY: Immediately after the death, they're more interested in the patient's pathology. They aren't interested in psychological issues.

SA: Now people are beginning to talk about it. They have got to work through their feelings somehow to be able to express them, because they really couldn't put them into words then. Probably there was some grief and depression.

AS: Despite the antagonism towards Mrs. Abel, did we pick up any feeling of grief or of real sadness about her death?

SY: The only persons who seemed to express it were two aides. They said it was sad, and had relatively nice things to say about her, and that you can't help but feel badly.

SY: I felt badly that the patient went, never having made peace with herself.

AS: You also felt badly because she was abandoned. But I'm not sure that that's grief. Do you sense that it is grief in whatever definition you would give of it? Have you felt grief before?

SY: No. I guess not.

SA: I have. A close friend. I certainly would equate the feeling that I had in intensity with what I felt for my friend. I sensed that the chaplain had—I don't know what you would call it—depression perhaps.

SY: I forget to say that I have learned the limits of how much I can tolerate a patient's talking about death and the anxieties that she goes through. Strange that as I was working with the patient, when she talked about dying, it didn't disturb me as much as with my two previous patients.

THEORETICAL COMMENTARY: THE LAST DAYS

Our commentary for this final section of Mrs. Abel's case rests mainly on the theories of "awareness context" and "dying trajectories" as developed in our two earlier books *(Awareness of Dying, and Time for Dying)*. During this phase of the lingering trajectory all relationships with and around Mrs. Abel continue to become attenuated or utterly collapse. Surgery as a last resort is a dramatic incident in her personal story, but is only the final event in the drama of her gradual, if not entirely total, insulation from personal and professional relationships with the staff.

The period comprising Mrs. Abel's last days and weeks began after Christmas vacation when the nursing staff became clearly aware that there was nothing more to do toward aiding the recovery of their patient. At this critical juncture in a dying trajectory the nursing staff usually shifts its intensive focus from managing a patient's pain to providing many other facets of comfort care—including painless comfort—appropriate to dying patients. This change to comfort care, and in the career provided by the hospital for implementing it, becomes then the general set of conditions under which a dying patient's last days unfold.

Mrs. Abel's last days and weeks themselves are characterized by several evolving courses of action. Some were initiated during the pain phase of her dying trajectory, and carried through until death. For instance, one was the staff nurses' intolerance of Mrs. Abel, which continued to grow, reaching the breaking point during these last weeks of her ordeal. The staff would settle only for her discharge to another ward, to surgery, or out of the hospital. Their only respite in the end was Mrs. Abel's death. Another carry-over was Dr. Colp's intense, personal concern for the management of Mrs. Abel's pain. This continued into the last days, thus he was disinclined to discharge her to the county hospital, or to a nursing home where her care might well be mismanaged. He personally became very involved in preventing her discharge. Yet removal to the county hospital is appropriate for such a lingering, indigent patient once she is in the nothing-more-to-do phase of dying, needing only comfort care, and is likely to live yet for some weeks. The result of the physician's concern was a collision course: the nursing staff pushed for a discharge and the doctor sidestepped it with every resource at his command. The collision ended in a nearly complete breakdown of communication between doctor and nurses. The social worker could only arrange, not actually bring about, the discharge. The solution to this dilemma was surgery, with two possible outcomes—either death or a change of wards with some measure of pain reduction for the patient (and perhaps even a later discharge). This could mean finally a discharge for the original nursing staff and a relinquishing of the patient's care by Dr. Colp.

Also carried over to this period of Mrs. Abel's dying trajectory was the student nurse's deepening involvement with Mrs. Abel, intensified by a concern over how poorly her last days were being managed. Mrs. Abel was becoming more and more isolated by the nursing staff and her doctor; gradually she was forced by them, in spite of her degenerating condition, to be more responsible for the decision to undergo neurosurgery. During this trying time Mrs. Abel herself became increasingly aware that she was dying and, indeed, would die relatively soon, with or without surgery. She always, however, continued to hold a glimmer of hope for a reprieve somehow from this dread destiny. Following in the path of this growing open awareness context among all participants to the trajectory was the chaplain who was trying to help Mrs. Abel prepare herself for death. His failure in giving Mrs. Abel religious consolation became more apparent the closer she came to the moment of surgery. The chaplain finally turned her over to a bewildered student-chaplain.

As the courses of action unfolded during the last days they influenced, intertwined, and combined with each other to result in the final outcome: a decision to try neurosurgery. This decision, so to speak, was not made but grew by default out of the combination of pressures from the various strands of evolving behavior. Once the decision had grown sufficiently to initiate preparations for surgery, its formulation was halted; so the purpose of surgery never was clearly understood by the patient, nursing staff, chaplain, doctor, social worker, student nurse or research nurse. At this juncture, the people surrounding Mrs. Abel made no effort to prevent the dubious surgery, and under various pretexts began to "pull out" of the situation completely. Only a few aides and the student remained close by to manage her last days. This nearly complete isolation forced Mrs. Abel to face an ominous fate alone, in pain, and with few resources beyond her own dark thoughts. Even the student, her last and best companion who helped her prepare for the surgery and possible death, failed (contrary to her promise) to arrive to comfort Mrs. Abel before surgery. Mrs. Abel went to the operating table rejected by all and shorn of her last pride and joy—her hair.

In the next pages we shall develop some of the conceptual details of these courses of action in an effort to explain why the last days of this lingering trajectory unfolded and ended as they did.

The most vital force shaping the end of Mrs. Abel's dying trajectory was the growing *intolerance* of the staff to her complaints of pain, her ritualistic demands during baths, meals, pain medication, and so forth, and her abiding need for companionship and attention which were further stimulated by the staff's avoidance of her. Generally, dying patients do not experience such intolerance by a nursing staff because they do not engender it by behavior such as Mrs. Abel's. Thus nursing staffs will usually be more concerned over not letting patients die alone, keeping them comfortable and informed, helping them prepare for death and settle affairs, and helping them through their last hours.

There were three major consequences of this intolerance for Mrs. Abel's last days. The first was the pressure the nursing staff put on Dr. Colp to *discharge* her. They thereby created a condition which forced him to list her as a research patient and then to send her to surgery, as ways of keeping her at the medical center. A further consequence of this conflict between the nurses and doctor was to reduce the effectiveness of Mrs. Abel's care, and the normal flow of information between them about her condition which Mrs. Abel's growing awareness demanded. Though the doctor thought her care was the best any hospital could provide, it fell far short of the best. The doctor's growing avoidance of the nurses prevented him from monitoring and realizing the kind of care and information that she actually received. The second consequence of the staff's intolerance was the growing *isolation* of Mrs. Abel. Again this reduced the calibre of her care. A third consequence was that the staff did not help Mrs. Abel *prepare* herself for death on a daily basis. The student and chaplain only partially filled this need.

A major consequence for the staff of their intolerance was, of

165

course, that the ward's sentimental order was continually in disarray. The nurses could barely discuss the case with each other. Nurses usually talk quite readily to help support each other during such ordeals. An effort by the supervisor to call a staff conference never jelled. Staff members could not or would not talk of the case to each other in any manner which would relieve them, and became intolerant of the student and fieldworker who wanted to discuss Mrs. Abel with them. In the end, forgetting of the dying patient was begun by avoiding her, and it ended by the staff never discussing her fate after she had died. The standard tactic for laying to rest a patient's story which is not too easily forgotten is to develop a post-mortem story. This explains away loose ends that prevent easy forgetting. This tactic was not used in Mrs. Abel's case.

The staff's intolerance of Mrs. Abel had a major consequence for the doctor: it drove him from the ward except for brief visits, mostly at night ,and forced him to resolve that he would never again bring a patient to this ward. Indeed he decided to return to research and give up the care of cancer patients per se. At one point, he tried to relinquish her case to the research physician, but the latter showed up in her room only once. Dr. Colp subsequently turned over her care to the neurosurgeons, who would only share it with him at the end of her life. They refused her admittance to their ward. His only "out" became surgery since he could not accept the idea of discharging her.

Mrs. Abel's last days began with the ward's sentimental order in a depressed state, verging on complete breakdown because of the growing intolerance of her. This intolerance was now coupled with the staff's awareness of impending death; meaning, of course, that they would have to manage it. The supervisor went into immediate action to shore up the sentimental order and solve the problem of Mrs. Abel. She applied various tactics to spread the burden of care, which we find in many dying situations when they have become an ordeal for the staff. "I am really more concerned about my staff than I am about Mrs. Abel," she told the fieldworker. She rotated girls constantly away from Mrs. Abel. She used float nurses—nurses brought in to help out on a ward—as much as she dared without fear of losing them, and she relegated as much care as possible to aides. The staff thought up ways of putting Mrs. Abel in a location so all could watch her without coming near—such as by a window readily seen from the nursing station. The supervisor, as well as staff, jumped at the chance to turn some of Mrs. Abel's care over to the student nurse. They said, "We should give her a medal for putting up with and taking care of Mrs. Abel." However, in the end they rejected the student because of her concern, care, and communication with Mrs.

Abel, which were in contrast to their unabiding intolerance and inadequacy in dealing with Mrs. Abel's talk about dying.

The supervisor and head nurse encouraged an "official face" of a happy and well organized staff concerned with the emotional well-being of Mrs. Abel. The supervisor defended, and apologized to Dr. Colp for, the staff's behavior as it leaked through this official "front": "They are doing the best job they can on Mrs. Abel." Dr. Colp, in turn, however, made no effort to release the steam behind the staff's intolerance by giving them some appreciation of what they did manage to accomplish with Mrs. Abel. This course of action readily led to conflict between staff and doctor in the every day care of Mrs. Abel on such basic issues as pain relief, baths, meals, and attention. It also led the supervisor to push for Mrs. Abel's discharge, without a direct request for this from the staff. The head nurse also pushed for discharge, and this effort lost no momentum despite the change of head nurse. In the staff's mind, a discharge, whether out of the hospital or transfer to another ward, was the only solution to the crushed sentimental order of their ward. A social worker eventually was all prepared to arrange the discharge in a feasible way as a tactic to force Dr. Colp to stop avoiding the issue with fears of house liens and typical "county" hospital care.

The chaplain wanted to start a team conference "to bring out guilt feelings" about Mrs. Abel in order to reinstate the sentimental order—a usual tactic in dying situations—but could not arrange the conference. A partial relief was meaningless to the staff, because nothing they did worked in controlling Mrs. Abel; for example, her temper. Therefore, nothing could reduce their frustration and helplessness except discharge. They could not listen to her talk about dying or death but rather could only say, "stop crying and eat. It doesn't help you." In short, the staff could not let her prepare for death on their time. They needed to be rid of her once and for all, irrespective of the consequences.

The patient's growing awareness of her fate contributed to the increasing intolerance of staff. Her growing need to prepare herself for death was cause for more rebuff. Mrs. Abel did find in the night nurse someone who would respond to her plea, "I want somebody to love me." The nurse, whose own mother had died of cancer, felt a reawakening of this personal loss and holding Mrs. Abel in her arms let her cry it out. But this form of comfort care so usual in dying situations was soon given up by this nurse. She too avoided and isolated Mrs. Abel, using the typical strategy of sending an aide into the room when Mrs. Abel called. The nurse wished also to heavily sedate Mrs. Abel but could not because of her slow respiraation. Mrs. Abel would awaken and scream at night, disturbing both other patients and the sentimental order of the ward. Clearly this unusually upsetting behavior had to be stopped, by discharging the patient.

The chaplain tried through prayer and a little religion to work with Mrs. Abel's expressed need to prepare for death. But he too could not take her crying when he found also that really there was "no communication" about religious matters. His suggestion that she take the attitude of "a courageous woman facing death" only ended in the failure of his effort. As Mrs. Abel told the one person who effectively helped her prepare for her fate, the student nurse, "I know more religion than he does." The student nurse let Mrs. Abel reminisce at will on prayer, her father, her marriage, her frustrating life, her beautiful hair, her intelligence, and her deformity in one leg. She let her pray at will with no interference. She helped fix her cherished hair, while the chaplain voiced doubts that Mrs. Abel really cared for her appearance. In short, the student helped her prepare for death in her own way, while the chaplain—despite his usual effectiveness with dying patients—could not, and the staff could allow hardly any terms at all.

One saving grace for the staff in Mrs. Abel's growing awareness was that she relaxed her control over pain management and eased up on her ritualistic demands. In now facing death, her attention was focusing on this as well as on pain. Preparations for death and dying claimed her thoughts. Also, physically she became less alert, and more lethargic and sleepy as her condition advanced. Instead of relaxing with this reduced stress, however, the staff nurses suspected that Mrs. Abel's intense pain was not really as intense as she had previously claimed. This paradox made them all the more intolerant of her "obnoxious" controls, demands, and complaints, in spite of their reduction.

At first the staff did not recognize the change in Mrs. Abel's personality which came about as a result of her growing awareness of dying. Finally they noticed this change, by the end of January when it became clear Mrs. Abel was worried about annoying them. For she felt her growing isolation. She then begged the staff, "Don't hate me," and acted more childish, submissive, and less talkative, and became still less demanding about controlling her pain. With unbending intolerance the staff still retreated, unyielding in their isolation of Mrs. Abel and in their remand that she be discharged. The psychological and social dimensions of comfort care, so often found in care of dying patients, was absent among these nurses because they could not sustain this kind of care with this particular patient. They had long ago lost the ability to give much more than physical care to her, and not entirely the best of that because of their withdrawal from her.

As January proceeded, with the staff, head nurse, supervisor, and social worker all pushing for discharge, Dr. Colp still would make no plans for discharge and, as we have said, he made fewer and briefer visits to the ward in order to avoid the nurses. The few visits he made, usually at night, entailed only the most perfunctory of communications with staff. The sentimental order of the ward was crumbling, with no discharge plans to bolster it.

To placate the staff, finally Dr. Colp noted on the chart that Mrs. Abel would be discharged after the pain research. This actually meant, as staff well knew, discharge after funds for the project ran out since these funds, not the research itself, were used by Dr. Colp as a tactic to delay discharge for financial reasons. His delaying tactic did not last long. The doctor in charge of pain research showed up only once, and never returned to Mrs. Abel. The research funds quickly ran out, and Dr. Colp was still in charge, while the staff relentlessly pushed for a discharge—if only a transfer to another ward. The supervisor, however, would not allow a transfer to any other ward.

The doctor in charge of pain research had, in passing, suggested a lobotomy. Dr. Colp explored this approach while continuing to delay Mrs. Abel's discharge. While inquiring into neurosurgery, Dr. Colp had to relay the well-conceived plan of the social worker for discharging Mrs. Abel to a nursing home on state funds. His tactic consisted of not grasping that her own home would require no lien, her savings not be soaked up, her husband not be financially wiped out. He forbade the sale of Mrs. Abel's car, the only obstacle to state aid. The social worker could not "reach" him. Later, a regular social worker when hearing about the physician's "irrationality" said she knew that Dr. Colp had trouble discharging all patients, a pattern which became extreme in Mrs. Abel's case. Dr. Colp also stated he felt the Medical Center owed Mrs. Abel some hospital care for her participation in research! This assertion left social workers and staff very upset. They tried to tell him that the Medical Center had carried Mrs. Abel, not vice versa, but Dr. Colp was too upset to comprehend.

Again Dr. Colp placated the nurses with a delaying tactic, noting on her chart, "If no surgery, discharge in a few weeks." This time he backed up the tactic with the additional notation, "If surgery is successful, discharge within eight to ten days." Thus, no matter what the outcome, including a third unnoted possibility of death, the delay had a resolution tacked on the end of it—no more Mrs. Abel—to underpin the ward's sentimental order and stop the nurs-

169

ing staff from immediately pushing for a discharge. The nurses' response was horror at the thought of a lobotomy, but silence at the thought of any protest. The thought of turning Mrs. Abel into a "vegetable" was hard to bear, though perhaps such a *social death* (ordinarily the consequence of natural causes rather than human action) would make it easier on the next staff which had to care for her than she currently was for themselves. The chaplain, too, was shocked by the thought of a lobotomy, previously having seen many such cases in a mental hospital, but he did not protest. The staff's extraordinary silence was accompanied by their giving Mrs. Abel virtually no information about or conception of what a lobotomy' meant, so she herself might adequately protest the operation.

Dr. Colp, too, was chary with any information to Mrs. Abel except to allude to the pain relief it might bring. All detailed questions were referred to the neurosurgeons. Clearly the various courses of action in which all these people engaged were converging toward a push—with no let up—in the direction of surgery. Nevertheless, the final decision was placed in the hands of Mrs. Abel! (Ordinarily the decision is up to the family or the patient, always in conjunction with the physician's best advice.) The conditions the physician and nurses created, and Mrs. Abel's own physical condition, forced her to confirm rather than rationally resolve the decision to undergo brain surgery. But Mrs. Abel did make an attempt at making a rational decision before her physical condition overcame her. Let us review her course of action during this trying period of decision making to see how it fed into the more general stream of social action, as the entire staff attempted to bring an end to her lingering on this ward (her hospital career) and perhaps to end her life (her dying trajectory).

Mrs. Abel's part in this drama can be divided into three stages related to her decision to undergo surgery: her behavior before the decision, during it, and then during the delay before surgery. Each stage was closely involved with her growing awareness of dying. Her initial awareness that she possibly was dying was based on *her* own interpretation of lasting pain and body degeneration. Only medication could reduce the pain, so obviously she must be getting no better. On the contrary, she was getting worse; her arms and legs were swelling with edema, and her cancer was slowly spreading. The realization that she might die led initially to a wish for the relief of death: "Please God do something. Either take me or make me feel better. I can't stand it, I want to die or be in a coma." She concluded finally that she wanted either to recover or die—and whichever, the sooner the better. In short, she became very ambivalent about whether or not to go on living.

These interpretations and feelings, so often managed to good effect by the nurses of dying patients, were ignored in this case by the staff. They made virtually no effort to help her to interpret and conclude her life in a manner that might relieve her anxiety nor did they help her prepare for the possible outcomes of living or dying. Rather they shut up her talk about death whenever they could not avoid her. As a result, her ambivalence about life and death grew stronger and edged toward the dying side, as her pain grew and as pain medication became less effective and had to be reduced because of difficulties in her respiration. The efforts of the student to discuss her dying with Mrs. Abel could not balance the deteriorating social conditions around the patient nor her worsening physical condition. She became a "set up" for making a ready confirmation of the suggestion to undergo surgery as a way to attain either painless life or death—although the suggestion was presented to her for a rational and responsible reply!

Nevertheless, Mrs. Abel did try to be rational and responsible. Ordinarily this would be an acceptable task for a patient with an alert mind. For her it was an enormous task, with the odds against her as a patient living under conditions of isolation, financial distress, pressure for her discharge, and because she was offered no other alternative than surgery to pain and physical degeneration. Mrs. Abel did as most patients do in such trying circumstances. She took a temporal view of the decision which was under consideration, and tried to gather information from staff and doctors to make the decision sensible. First she tried to find out how long she would probably last with and without surgery, and in what possible physical condition in either case. Would she die soon without surgery? If not, could they control the pain until she died? With surgery would she die soon or live on, pain free, for an appreciably long time? If she did live on would it be as a "vegetable" or with her usually alert mind? Also, how long should she hold out with or without surgery for a possible new cure? Thus she was trying to balance the alternative probabilities for death or a life with or without a social death. The staff would give no information to her on her condition either now or for the foreseeable future, and they would not discuss the lobotomy and its possible consequences. Dr. Colp would only say that the surgery was to reduce pain, and reduce pain, and referred Mrs. Abel to the surgeons for all details. He also implied that there was nothing else anyone could do for her. Thus he eliminated alternative paths, especially that of going directly to the nursing home. While this withholding of information was occurring, both doctor and staff delayed her current, daily care more and more. Without information and under stress, her temporal view was totally uncertain and her decision indecisive from the standpoint of reasonable choice.

But Mrs. Abel took the "responsibility" and agreed to the surgery under the pressure of the foregoing social and physical circumstances. Her fear of being turned into a vegetable could not balance fear of continued pain. Death was preferable only because now it was more probable than recovery. Even the student evaded her questions about the feasibility of surgery, principally so as not to interfere with the staff and doctors who were the people responsible for Mrs. Abel's hospital career. The surgeons did reduce Mrs. Abel's anxiety somewhat by assuring her that reduction in pain would most likely be one benefit of an operation. Mrs. Abel agreed to it. Surgery was then ordered.

The surgery was an unusual one at this hospital and required preparations that were not readily met. Tests had to be made on the patient. Instruments had to be ordered and repaired. Meanwhile Dr. Colp was out of town. This was not his specialty. The doctor, found to do the operation, wanted to practice up on a procedure that he was developing called a hyperphysectomy. The purpose of the operation itself was never clarified beyond the notion of tumor reduction. The kaleidoscope of reasons for the surgery for staff, Dr. Colp, and Mrs. Abel did not require much clarification.

These preparations and procedural decisions took time that resulted for all parties in an *agonizing delay* before surgery. The waiting forced a renewed, agonizing interplay of the nurses still pushing for some kind of discharge, the doctor still needing to keep Mrs. Abel in the hospital, the student still trying to understand the care of dying and this patient in particular, and Mrs. Abel still demanding pain relief, information, attention, and trying to handle her ambivalence about surgery and death as her awareness of how long she might live was sharpened by her physical deterioration. The delay thereby forced an even greater isolation of Mrs. Abel as everyone evaded her more or pulled away completely, feeling that the surgery just over the horizon was their resolution to an impossible patient. Let us consider how these particular (and unusual) courses of intertwining action proceeded during this delay in surgery.

During the delay Mrs. Abel's physical condition deteriorated rapidly, with several consequences for all concerned. She became incontinent. Her edema increased to the point where fluid oozed from her leg. Her respiration was very depressed; her lethargy and sleep increased. This latter condition made Mrs. Abel even more unmanageable when awake. She had tantrums, screamed, wept un-

172

controllably, demanded pain medication, and resorted to her former rituals of controls. There was, in short, a distinct personality change occurring which made her even more difficult or obnoxious to staff, doctor, and chaplain. The student nurse stood by her almost to the last, against Dr. Colp's advice to avoid her and quit her death talk.

Mrs. Abel's lethargy and sleep further indicated to the nursing staff that she really did not have as much pain as she had tried to convince them. Otherwise, how could she sleep so much? They became even more disgusted with her efforts at managing her pain medication. She was devalued further for at last they had clear evidence. Dr. Colp still defended her pain intensity.

Because she sank faster than expected problems were created about the forthcoming surgery. Mrs. Abel's awareness made her now wonder if she would die before reaching the table rather than on it! The meaning of her "Please God, I want to die" changed. She began begging for surgery "today," clearly wishing to end her life and suffering as soon as possible (a kind of suicide) on the table, yet she still clung to the faint hope of a miracle from the surgery.

From day to day she was never informed when the surgery was rescheduled or why it was continually postponed, and why pain medication was withheld more and more. This isolation literally forced her to crave surgery all the more. The student tried to explain to her the delay when she was stunned to find out that Mrs. Abel knew of none of the problems attending the forthcoming operation. In response to the blood and respiration problems, Mrs. Abel said, "What difference does it make, I'm going to die anyway." She had reached the point where such explanations meant little in view of her awareness of death. The student, left with "picking up the pieces," could only try to prepare her with current information for more delay.

The student herself became very upset with the delay and with Mrs. Abel's isolation before the surgery. She listened to Mrs. Abel, held her hand, bathed her body. She could not stand the notion of Mrs. Abel dying alone because her own father had faced sudden death alone. The staff grew to dislike the student increasingly for taking over the burden of Mrs. Abel. The student continued with the death talk in which Mrs. Abel engaged in order to reconcile herself to death. Finally, when surgery was definitely scheduled, Mrs. Abel wanted to be sure the student would be with her the day before the operation. However, the student could not come and Mrs. Abel desperately offered her money to come. The student promised to come the following day just before surgery, in consolation; but, as we know, she never arrived. Mrs. Abel's isolation before surgery was complete.

The student felt terrible about not showing up but acknowledged she slept late to avoid seeing Mrs. Abel's precious hair shaven off and her being wheeled off to surgery. The situation had become, in the end, too much even for her. She also felt that the surgeons really would not do surgery after all because of Mrs. Abel's very poor condition. Obviously in rationalizing her non-appearance, she underestimated the push toward surgery from nursing staff and attending doctor. The student also realized, as helpless as she was to do something, that in the end she had done as much as humanly possible by trying to give Mrs. Abel considerable attention, comfort, and understanding. This was, of course, considerably more than the staff, doctor, chaplain, and social worker had managed to give the patient. How Mrs. Abel lived as she died during these last few days was thus a responsibility that only the student tried to shoulder or succeeded in carrying. In many dying situations we have observed, nursing staff does take on this responsibility and succeed in their efforts.

By the time Mrs. Abel was scheduled for surgery, Dr. Colp knew she was running a race with death. He realized it was only a matter of days before she would, without the surgery, slip into a comatose state. However, he left the responsibility and risk of surgery up to the neurosurgeons, while he made Mrs. Abel responsible for getting information from the surgeons so as to make her own decision about surgery. The doctor wanted to cover himself against a possible lawsuit, because Mrs. Abel had been known to sue hospitals before. Yet in switching this responsibility to other shoulders, he continued to push for surgery.

First he told Mrs. Abel he wanted her to make up her mind for sure, because to change her mind at the last minute might upset the surgeons! Second, after his pre-operation examination, he did not mention the fluid in Mrs. Abel's chest to the neurosurgeons. All told, he felt his findings did not really matter; but if he reported them, the surgery might be forestalled because of the risk in the surgeon's minds. The surgeons proceeded with the operation accepting, without details, his judgment that she could undergo surgery. After her death the surgeons would not say that this one additional condition had caused her death but rather that there were a complex of causative conditions. Dr. Colp felt that his withholding of his findings was only a calculated risk, not an error of judgment or communication. His calculated risk was taken to resolve through surgery the pressures on him to do something about Mrs. Abel's discharge, her pain, and her financial status.

The nursing staff was pleased with his persistence about surgery, though they could hardly believe the surgeons would perform it on a patient in Mrs. Abel's condition. Yet, their guilt was not strong enough to cause them to protest the surgery, they wanted Mrs. Abel off the ward so much. Dr. Colp later told the staff he did not blame them for their treatment of Mrs. Abel toward the end. He assured them he would have discharged her a month ago except for his decision to try a lobotomy. Thus he pulled away from Mrs. Abel, showing them that at last he was on their side.

In spite of trying to make these amends to the ward's sentimental order, he privately vowed never to have a patient on this floor again and told the staff he would return to full time research. Thus it disturbed him considerably in the last days when the student persisted in caring for Mrs. Abel, but he tried to act as if he no longer was concerned. He told the student that he had "washed his hands" of Mrs. Abel and that, "You really don't have to go in to see her." The student saw through his pretended disinvolvement.

We know from Chapter II what happened to Mrs. Abel. We now have some idea of the intertwining of courses of action that led to her death. The certainty and time of her death had been predicted, quite accurately by Dr. Colp when she entered the hospital in November. The staff and patient had to develop the temporal and certainty expectations of her trajectory on their own because the doctor told no one of his expectations. At the end the awareness context was open and clear on both certainty and time of death. At no point in Mrs. Abel's lingering trajectory could her dying and death have been averted by medical science.

The only *change* that could have been made in this tragic trajectory was in the life that Mrs. Abel had to live while dying. We know from our studies of dying in hospitals that Mrs. Abel could have had a considerably more compatible hospital career. The first step to insure compatible hospital careers for dying patients is the training of nurses and physicians in psychological and sociological understanding of dying patients and of themselves in relation to a dying patient.* This training should be linked with an understanding of the impact of hospital organization on professionals' care of dying patients. In Chapter V we present our comments on useful ways to help manage a dying patient's trajectory.

---

*See our recommendations in *Time for Dying* (Chicago: Aldine Publishing Company, 1968) pp 251 - 260 and Jeanne C. Quint, Anselm L. Strauss, and Barney G. Glaser, "Improving Nursing Care of the Dying," *Nursing Forum*, Vol. VI, No. 4 (1967), pp. 368-78.

CHAPTER V

COMMENTS: THEORETICAL and PRACTICAL

While neglected in recent years the case history, we believe, still remains an enterprise of great merit for sociology. In giving prominence to the story for its own sake, a case history may still contribute to theory and practice. One needs not always engage in a case study with its analytic purpose and constructions to make such contributions. In this chapter we briefly review how a case study may in several ways contribute to theory and practice.

THEORETICAL CONTRIBUTIONS

Through a case history, explained and interpreted by theoretical commentary, the sociologist can describe in detail a theoretically important type,[1] average, extreme, or exemplar case.[2] The dense, readable imagery provided by the case history allows further development of an important aspect of the general theory. It, in effect starts initiating a sub-theory, such as one on lingering hospitalized dying in Mrs. Abel's case. While lingering is only one of many aspects of

---

[1]

For example, the professional thief. See Edwin H. Sutherland, *The Professional Thief,* (Chicago, Illinois: The University of Chicago Press, 1937).

[2]

An exemplar is the case that exemplifies that average or majority of cases. See David Matza, *Delinquency and Drift,* (New York: John Wiley and Sons, Inc., 1964).

dying in hospitals or at home, it is an increasingly prevalent and important aspect of dying, requiring both more research and more theoretical understanding and explanation.

This sub-theory on a socially prevalent problem easily leads to its formation as an *applicable* sociological theory. This formation appears to be a two step process. First the sociologist shows how well a theory or theories may usefully and relevantly explain and interpret a single case history from a sociological perspective. Second, in showing sociologists, other professionals and laymen how well the theory works, the sociologists also shows how well it can be used on other single cases for understanding and possibly controlling some of them. If readers actually are engaged in the area [are working (nurses of lingering patients), or have dealings (family members of lingering patients)] then they now will have theory to apply in coping with their own working situations. Thus in contribution to the development of applied social theory, case histories help solve an important task facing sociological theory today.

Generating and verifying theory is such an abstract activity that often people try to comprehend the theory for their own use, (as in teaching, research or actual application) without sufficient understanding either of the phenomenon from which the theory came and for which it may be used. While very specific in relation to the theory, a case history with commentary delineating its theoretical context and meaning tends to give readers, through its dense imagery, a fuller and deeper comprehension of the theory. The theory for these people becomes less abstract, less reified, and more pertinent to reality. This is especially so for a formal theory that has never, seldom, or long since been grounded or related to data. A theory which, for example, people know how and why to use, will probably be used more often, with more relevance. This use in turn will serve to increase the theory's longevity as a viable sociological theory.

A case history also provides a vehicle for the integration of several theories at different levels. This grounded tie-in of theories makes their integration meaningful since it carries the resulting composite theory to a more general level. For example, one can say we have approached in this particular case study a more general theory of dying since we have welded together our theories of awareness of dying, dying trajectories and pain management in commenting on this case.

In applying a theory to a case history one gets a measure of feedback, as with all data, that contributes to cleaning up and rounding out of the theory. This feedback tends to force clarification of the theory's categories and hypotheses. It tends to systematize integration of the theory, and it tends to increase the theory's density at various levels of generality as the analyst finds himself generating new ideas from the case history to fill in gaps in the theory. It delimits the scope of the theory by showing how much of the materials of the case can and cannot be handled by the theory, and it suggests areas within the theory which require further research and development through additional generation and verification.

PRACTICAL CONTRIBUTIONS

The reader could not have read the foregoing chapters without drawing the conclusion that it has radical implications for changing and perhaps improving the nursing and medical care given to the dying. Mrs. Abel's case, of course, has highlighted several problems of terminal care—but we caution against too hasty a criticism based on this single case. Its contribution is merely to highlight extant problems of a general nature (which exist in a multitude of similar cases), and indicate the theory that may be used to cope with these problems. The generality of some of the problems attendant to Mrs. Abel's case and the context within which they occur have been shown in our other books on dying.[3]

In Time for Dying we made four recommendations toward improving the care of dying patients based on our theory of dying.[4] These recommendations, to be sure, imply a critique of current practices, many of which are found in Mrs. Abel's case. They were offered as a set of related recommendations, each bearing on the other. The systematic nature of our theoretical commentary on Mrs. Abel's case allows a highlighting of how these recommendations apply in one instance—which additionally suggests their importance in guiding the first steps of a general reform of terminal care. The goal of such a reform—by almost anyone's standards—is to improve the current system on the social-psychological level in order to make terminal care more compassionate and more effective vis-a-vis patients as social and psychological beings.

---

[3]
Awareness of Dying and *Time for Dying*, (Aldine Publishing Co., 1965) (Aldine Publishing Co., 1968); Also *The Nurse and the Dying Patient*, (New York: MacMillan Co., 1967), Jeanne Quint.

[4]
IBID., pp. 251-260.

1. *Training for giving terminal care should be greatly amplified and deepened in schools of medicine and nursing.*

The training that physicians and nurses receive as students equips them principally for restricted technical aspects of dealing with dying and death. Nothing is taught that explicitly helps them to understand and cope with the web of social relationships that grows up around a patient who lingers while dying. Of course this web is not always so disastrous for the patient as in Mrs. Abel's case. This web should be consciously understood by staff no matter what direction it take, so that a patient's social and psychological needs may be attended to in some measure and surely not inadvertently bruised in the name of technical requirements.

Mrs. Abel's situation highlights the clear implication that along with techniques in medical and nursing care, curricula in medical and nursing schools should be changed to include the more psychological, social and organizational aspects of terminal care. Our research and this case history suggest that extensive changes are needed for this education. Considerable experimentation will be necessary before faculties can be satisfied that they have provided adequate training in these aspects of terminal care. Clearly we cannot assume this training already exists even in the most advanced nursing schools attached to medical centers, as Mrs. Abel's case shows.

2. *Explicit planning and review should be given to the psychological, social and organizational aspects of terminal care.*

Although nursing and medical staff are well aware of the particular patterns of technical terminal care provided for the characteristic modes of dying on each type of ward—for example the kind of care provided a lingering patient, such as Mrs. Abel, on a cancer ward—they take very little cognizance in the planning and review of related matters that are not strictly "nursing" or "medical." Usually it takes a family member or a particularly sensitive nurse to force psychological, social or organizational issues on the staff's attention.

One clearly needed corrective for this situation is to make staff accountable for the many social and psychological actions toward the patient which are currently left to personal discretion and seldom, incidently reported.[5] Mrs. Abel's case clearly highlights the disastrous turn these actions may take when left to private initiative

---

5

"The Nonaccountability of Terminal Care," from *Hospitals*, Vol. 38, January 16. 1964.

and judgement and especially when negative actions finally become collectivized and supported by a group of nurses.

Being held accountable for the social and psychological aspects of their acts can begin at anytime for staff. But this accountability will be more useful when staff become trained in understanding what is happening socially, psychologically and organizationally to themselves, the patient and the family.

It would have helped Mrs. Abel a great deal if the nurses were held psychologically and socially accountable for their treatment of her to someone whose understanding could have forestalled her consequent isolation and avoidance. It would have helped Mrs. Abel even more if the nurses themselves had been trained in the necessary insights that would give them some deeper understanding of Mrs. Abel's demands and their own distress, so they could have responded to her needs beneficially while controlling their own annoyance.

Once the staff is familiar with understandings of the social and psychological needs of dying patients, they can begin organizing the work of the ward to include these needs in their care of patients. The hospital can develop organizational supports to backstop the nurses and doctors in such difficult circumstances. The availability of a chaplain, such as we found in Mrs. Abel's case, is one such support. Specially trained nurses to handle difficult dying cases as Mrs. Abel can be made available. Every now and then they emerge on their own and other nurses turn to them. New organizational mechanisms must be invented to handle dying within the context of the organization.

3. *There should be explicit social-psychological planning for phases of the dying trajectory that occur before and after residence at the hospital.*

Most planning for phases outside the hospital is strictly medical, or deals with financial aspects of the patient's life or with matters of geographic mobility. This planning usually lacks a consideration of these feelings and needs of patients or their families. This sort of planning would have been strategic in Mrs. Abel's case. The hospital was not systematically set-up for devising a reasonable plan for getting Mrs. Abel out of the hospital. Merely sending her to county hospital would have meant financial ruin for her and her husband by having a lien put against their house. This was unacceptable to her doctor. When the social worker finally found state funds to put her in a nursing home, this was still unacceptable to him regarding what he felt was the type of medical and nursing care she would receive. The doctor's only alternative was to keep her in the hospital on research funds. There could, for example, be a county health office charged with helping to plan adequate terminal care and the kind of "tender-loving-care" a patient needs when dying outside the hospital.

4. *Finally, medical and nursing personnel should encourage public discussion of issues that transcend professional responsibilities for terminal care.*

This recommendation refers to certain events that repeatedly occur during dying trajectories and are debated by hospital personnel. These events represent grave problems such as the withholding of addicting drugs, and the senseless prolonging of life— especially when it entails undue agony for the patient and family and/or financial ruin for the remaining family. These problems are genuinely unresolvable by the professional community, because they belong in the public domain. Only when they are debated within the wider public arena, so that sentiment develops for certain solutions, can hospital personnel begin to act in genuinely rational ways with public support about these problems.

These grave problems did affect Mrs. Abel adversely. Her dying would have been less stressful if the nurses had been more rational and understanding about her drugs, if the doctor had been more clearly guided by public policy and sentiment on undue prolonging and financial ruin. Mrs. Abel's agony was in some measure due to lack of clear alternatives to these problems supported by the community at large.

In conclusion, Mrs. Abel's case highlights for all concerned the necessity of beginning to solve many of the social-psychological problems of dying in hospitals. We offer our interrelated *set* of general recommendations as a first step in guiding the improvement of terminal care.

CHAPTER VI

CASE HISTORIES AND CASE STUDIES

This is a *case history*. It consists of a *story* about a lingering dying trajectory, along with an accompanying *theoretical commentary* about this story. To distinguish a case history from a case study as types of sociological enterprise is essential. In this chapter therefore, we shall discuss several distinguishing properties of case histories and studies from two vantage points: (1) the focus and purpose of each, and (2) the use and source of theory of each. We shall emphasize the case history approach to make clear what we have intended by this book. Also, we wish very much to stimulate the publication of case histories. They have passed out of fashion in sociology, although they still retain illustrative and pedagogic uses at least in psychology and anthropology.

THE FOCUS OF CASE HISTORIES

The focus of a case history is a full story of some temporal span or interlude in social life—a biography, an occupational career, a project, an illness, an evolution, a disaster, a ceremony, an evolvement, and so forth. The story is about *one social unit*—such as a person, a status, an organization, a process, a type of behavior, a relationship, a group, or a nation.

Many published cases have taken the form of "life histories,"[1] but they can be about other social phenomena. The theme of a case history, for instance, can be an occupational career, as in Suther-

---

1. W. I. Thomas and F. Znaniecki, *The Polish Peasant in Poland and America* (New York: Alfred A. Knopf, 1918).

land's book on the professional thief,[2] although the career may be secondary to a particular phase or phases in the career, as in Warner's case study of the rise and fall of a local political hero.[3] A case history may have as its major theme the evolution of family relations;[4] the total span of a lengthy, complicated public ceremony;[5] the events that follow a precipitation of an imaginary disaster;[6] or the evolving pattern of events after an actual disaster.[7] There is no reason why long case histories could not have other temporal themes: the evolution of relationship between business firms or among other organizations, the evolution of an organizational crisis or the breakdown of a battalion's morale.[8]

The research goal in a case history, then, is to get the fullest possible story *for its own sake*. In contrast, the case study is focused on analytic abstractions and constructions for purposes of description, or verification and/or generation of theory.[9] There is no attempt at obtaining the fullest possible story for its own sake. Fullness of description refers only to what data is needed for the constructions designated by the abstract purposes of the researcher. Of course, verification and generation of theory require even less data on the full story than a description requires. In sum, the case history gives prominence to the story—and to the "story line"—whereas in the case study the story is subordinated to abstract purpose.

In the case study, single or multiple cases are used, since the process of analytic abstracting-out eliminates any confusion over the various stories behind the different cases. Indeed, multiple cases

2. Edwin H. Sutherland, *The Professional Thief* (Chicago, Illinois: The University of Chicago Press, 1937).

3. W. L. Warner, *The Living and the Dead* (New Haven: Yale University Press, 1959), pp. 9-100.

4. Oscar Lewis, *The Children of Sanchez* (New York: Vintage Books, 1961).

5. W. L. Warer, *op. cit.*

6. Leon Festinger, Henry W. Reichen, and Stanley Schachter, *When Prophecy Fails* (Minneapolis, Minnesota: University of Minnesota Press, 1956).

7. L. Schatzman, *Community Reaction to Disaster*, Ph. D. Thesis, Indiana University, 1960.

8. Tamotsu Shibutani, *Improvised News: A Sociological Study of Rumor* (Indianapolis: The Bobbs-Merrill Company, Inc., 1966), see Chapter 5, pp. 129-63.

9. See, for example, in the same Bobbs-Merrill series ibid., on advanced studies in the social sciences, Alvin W. Gouldner and Richard A. Peterson, *Technology and the Moral Order* (1963), Julius Roth, *Timetables* (1963), and Fred Davis, *Passage Through Crisis* (1964).

are the requisite basis of broader generalities which are derived from comparisons. In contrast, most case histories have been and probably will be about single cases. Nevertheless, it is possible to do multiple case histories. These can be done under two conditions. First, each case is short enough so the book-length case history is not excessive Typically, case histories, because of the focus on the full story, are quite long. Second, the analyst has a theory that integrates the multiple case histories together in his commentary. Otherwise he has only a series of single case histories .

To achieve this theoretical integration, he can sample theoretically for his case histories.[10] This means that if he has a case history, and a theory to explain and interpret it then he can decide—on theoretical grounds—about other possible case histories that would provide good contrasts and comparisons. For example, our case history of Mrs. Abel, a hospital dying trajectory, might well be compared to a "recovering" trajectory in a tuberculosis hospital: thus we would be comparing two kinds of hospital careers. The resulting comparative analysis is different from that used in case studies for description, verification, or generation. In the case studies, one analyzes similarities and differences to establish empirical generalizations and variations and to verify and generate theory.[11]

Case histories, particularly long ones, seem to have declined in favor among sociologists, largely because of the advances in research methods which have supported the analytic and abstract thrust of the discipline. In spite of this neglect, sociologists continue to incorporate case histories as data within their case studies, and sometimes a case study itself is actually a case history. These stories embedded in data of a study may be short or long, consist of pure and unedited interviews or field notes or may be slightly constructed from the data because of the researcher's abstract orientation. The stories are not likely to be as full as the stories yielded by purposeful case history collection of data, but may be sufficiently full to be rendered as a case history. The fullest are more likely to be found within single book-length case studies. For example, in *Doomsday Cult* we have the story of the rise and failure of a "far-out" religious group.[12] Mrs. Abel's story was a lucky "find" on our part which occurred while we were collecting data for and publishing a study of dying in hospitals.

10. Barney G. Glaser and Anselm L. Strauss, *The Discovery of Grounded Theory* (Chicago: Aldine Publishing Company, 1967), Chapter 3, pp. 45-79.

11. *Ibid.,* Chapter 2, pp. 21-45.

12. John Lofland (Englewood Cliffs: Prentice-Hall, Inc., 1966).

Our point is that these case histories are collected by chance and sensitivity, but many are unpublished, or lie buried within case studies, and are destined never *per se* to see the light of day because sociologists today are not doing case histories. We say, "Look there may be a good story in your study, why not write it also." We wish researchers to review their materials for such stories and publish them—the more varied the better.

In view of the focus on analytic abstraction in current sociological work, it is perhaps preferable to do the research analysis first. Once this responsibility is off the researcher's chest, he can then enjoy the fun of writing a case history of his data. Also at this juncture he has the advantage of knowing or having discovered a theory from the research by which to comment on and explain the case history. An obvious alternative—and more efficient—is purposively to collect case histories from the start with the intent of writing them up, whether this collection is done along with a case study or as the sole purpose.

In and of itself, the case history is an enterprise of great merit in sociology. One need not always do an abstract study. Through a story, which is *explained and interpreted with theory, the sociologist* can show a type, an average, an extreme or an exemplar case. The case history then provides a very dense, readable imagery for sociological theory. (Currently, novelists much more than sociologists take on this task, but for their own purposes and with much less explicit theory. Their theory is also less integrated and frequently less complex than we would wish for sociological purposes.) A sociologists can show how well a theory may work by usefully and relevantly taking apart a single case history from a sociological view. This is the beginning of developing adequate *applied* social theory, an important task facing sociology today. A case history becomes a way of showing laymen how our theory might be used on single cases—possibly on their own case. From the history, people can gain much understanding of general phenomena through its theoretical interpretation and explanation.

This task of doing a case history is at one end of the continuum of abstraction in sociological work. At the other end is the generation of theory by multiple case studies and comparative analysis. (Between are the studies which involve descriptions and verifications, the former being closer to case histories.) *The fullest understandings of social phenomenon come, we believe, from dense case histories on one end of the continuum and from densely generated grounded theories on the other end of the continuum.* In between we have shredded, abstract descriptions; puzzle solving of portions of the theory; and verifications of portions of the fuller understandings found at either end of the continuum.

THEORY AND CASE HISTORIES

We turn now to a discussion of the relation of theory to case histories. For the most part, theory is *applied* to case histories in separate commentaries which explain and interprets parts of the story, as we have done in this book. These commentaries usually appear after each section of the story. Though undoubtedly it will happen, generating new theoretical notions from the story is only a by-product, not the main purpose of a case history. As for the reader, his typical tempo of reading is probably first to read the story, then the commentary, then reread the story for a greater understanding of it. The theoretical purposes of case studies, in contrast, are to generate and verify theory, with parts of the story being selectively interwoven with the theory as evidence and illustration.

Some case histories are published with virtually no theoretical commentary. This occurs when the author assumes that his readers are so familiar with a current theory that they can explain and interpret his case history without guidance. For example, in life histories published by anthropologists, often the reader is assumed to be familiar with anthropological theory and so can intelligently interpret the story without guidance. Similarly, Howard Becker has remarked—in introducing a new edition of Clifford Shaw's *The Jack-roller*[13]—that when this classic life history was first published sociologists read it as a piece of a large "mosaic" made up of the many sociological publications then issuing from the University of Chicago. Hense little explicit theoretical commentary was necessary for the readers of this case study. When only a little theoretical commentary accompanies a case history, generally it will appear at least in the beginning and end of the case, and refers the reader to a current theory that applies.

We shall discuss next those case histories requiring or accompanied by considerable theoretical commentary and analysis. What theory should be used for these case histories? The answer is: a theory which fits and is relevant to the data of the history. We suggest therefore that it be a theory grounded in the data of a substantive or a formal area to which the case history belongs. Logically-deducted theory based on speculations and assumptions seldom does justice to a case history and is very likely to distort the story. In our

---

13. (Chicago: The University of Chicago Press, 1967).

book, Mrs. Abel's story was analyzed with theory grounded in our study of dying in hospitals. Thus we shall apply our substantive and formal theories on dying to her case. They work very well. This reflects back on the usefulness of grounded theory: generating theory from the data of systematic research. However, sometimes the theory to be applied is formulated only on a formal level, as when psychiatrists utilize psychiatric theory to interpret a life history, (say, of a suicide) [14] or as when Sutherland discusses the life and occupation of a professional thief using the general sociological theory of occupations and culture current in his day. Another example is that the story of a person's rise in the military can be commented upon in terms of a grounded formal theory of organizational careers.[15] Thus case histories will vary in accordance with the level of generality of the theory or theories applied. The author must, of course, use the level of generality best suited to bringing out what he deems are essentials of his case history.

To be sure, the author need not use only one theory for his commentary. He can use several theories at different levels, provided he is clear about their individual use. For example, with Mrs. Abel we used our substantive theories on managing pain and dying trajectories[16] and our formal theory of awareness contexts.[17] This led to multiple interpretations and explanations at certain points, but main ly the theories were used successively. In contrast, case studies are usually devoted to one theory, with the exception of some description that use multiple, theoretical ways of describing an area. Since the theory (or theories) is applied to the case history, presumably it already exists. If none applicable exists, whether formal or substantive, then one can be generated for the task by the researcher.

An adequate method is to generate a substantive theory from the class of substantive data to which the story belongs. One cannot generate, however, an adequate theory *solely* from the case history itself. The theory would be too thin and unqualified: many cases are necessary for the comparative analysis that will yield a sufficiently dense and integrated substantive theory.[18] The several cases need,

---

14. Cf. the comments by Jack Douglas in his, *Social Meanings of Suicide* (Princeton: Princeton University Press, 1968), pp. 258-64.

15. See Barney G. Glaser (ed.), *Organizational Careers: A Sourcebook for Theory* (Chicago. Aldine Publishing Company, 1968).

16. Barney G. Glaser and Anselm L. Strauss, *Time for Dying* (Chicago: Aldine Publishing Company, 1968).

17. Barney G. Glaser and Anselm L. Strauss, *Awareness of Dying* (Chicago: Aldine Publishing Company, 1965).

18. See *Discovery of Grounded Theory, op cit.*, Chapter 6, pp. 117-61 for a discussion of integration and density of theory with respect to several studies.

however, only be studied sufficiently for generating theory. As we have shown in the *Discovery of Grounded Theory,* the amount of material needed for generating theory on each case may be very limited compared to a full history. The resulting substantive theory may be written "on its own" in an article, but also can be developed in the theoretical commentary made on a case history. A small amount of substantive theory can go a long way in explaining a case history. The research and generation may go fairly fast. To arrive at his theory, however, the analyst should be prepared to take as much time as needed.

The purpose of a theoretical commentary in explaining and in-preting the case history is to give a broadened picture of the parti-cular case. *The theory puts the case within a more general context of understanding what could have happened under varying condi-tions, and therefore why it happened this way within this particular case.* The particulars of the case, then, are interpreted generally as "what actually happened" within a range of several probabilities and alternatives. No longer can the case history be considered sim-ply as a typical exemplar or an idiosyncratic occurence, as is the tendency when the reader does not know the general perspective afforded by the theory. In contrast, the authors of case studies strive for generalization and testing theory and the story is a means to those ends. In case histories, theory is in the service of generalization and specifying the story context by placing it within a theoretical con-text and is best done, as noted earlier, when the theory is compara-tive.

To achieve this general understanding of a case history, some stylistic aspects of the theoretical commentary are clear to us now. Primarily, the analyst must use his theory selectively; that is, he uses only those parts of his theory that are most relevant to bring out a general understanding of the case. This requires mastery of the whole theory, and sensitivity in choosing its diverse possible applications to the case. Also, in developing the commentary the story is kept paramount and the theory subdued, although the theory prescribes what aspects of the total story will appear in the com-mentary. In short, the theoretical analysis is kept implicit through-out a running commentary on the story. In contrast, in case studies the emphasis is on making the theory explicit and structured.

THEORETICAL COMMENTARY IN EXISTING CASE HISTORIES AND STUDIES

In the sociological literature today only a thin line distinguishes most case histories from case studies, if they are distinguishable at all. There are few clear examples of case histories, like Sutherland's *The Professional Thief*. Most monographs and articles, particularly descriptive studies, have bits of case histories woven into them which function in the service of the researcher's more abstract purposes. Thus, what we have today mainly is a matter of degree in differentiating case studies from histories. Let us analyze some of these case studies to see what they can tell us also about the style and potentials of theoretical commentary in case history analysis.

Whether a case study is long or short, it is important to ask how the author writes his theoretical commentary into the publication. Among the relevant dimensions are: the *amount* of theory, its *level* of generality, its *source*, its degree of *systematization*, and the *density* with which it is formulated. We have already commented upon amount, source, and level of theory used in case histories. A few brief comments on systemization and density in case studies will suffice for understanding our ensuing analysis. In some case studies, the theoretical commentary is well wrought, nicely integrated—it "hangs together" systematically.[19] On the other hand, some theoretical commentaries are decidedly "loose," consisting merely of a collection of theoretical statements because little systematization is attempted. Theoretical commentary also may exhibit degrees of density. The theory may be "thin" (although systematically stated); whereas some theoretical commentary is densely detailed at several levels of generality and gives readers a sense of "depth" or rich context, whether or not the theory is relatively systematized.

With these five dimensions of theory in mind, one can usefully characterize the theoretical commentary of any case study *or* history *with some preciseness*. We emphasize the preceding phrase because ordinarily their functions are thought of in very general terms— what they illustrate, yield understanding of, or give evidence for sometimes is even left understated. The question however is: illustration, understanding or evidence for *what?* If we combine the five dimensions of theory, we have 32 cells by which to characterize the commentary. Thus a case might fall into a cell representing a theoretical commentary that is considerable in amount, highly generalized, systematic, dense, and drawn from outside the body of data which yielded the case. Psychoanalytic commentary about phychiatric "cases" is of this type. Our case history of Mrs. Abel falls into a cell representing theoretical commentary that is considerable in amount, substantive, systematic, dense, and is theory formulated by the authors from research in the same substantive areas to which the

---

19. Cf., Howard Becker, Blanche Geer, Everett C. Hughes, Anselm Strauss, *Boys In White* (Chicago: University of Chicago Press, 1962).

case pertains. We commented less, however, than would have been necessary if two volumes on dying had not previously been published by us. A case study like Festinger's[20] utilizes theory that is general and systematic, with the virtual exclusion of substantive theory about sectarian behavior because the senior researchers were intent on verifying a systematic general theory.

Sometimes a case study may fall into more than one cell. For instance, a case study of Bostonian Italians by Herbert Gans uses both general theory drawn from outside his research and substantive theory which emerged from his research.[21] The same technique for locating long cases can be used with short cases—the latter can be used to illustrate, for example, a general or substantive theory or an item of either type of theory. The commentary can be systematic or not, dense or not, drawn from outside the research or from its research data.

Stylistic features of cases (study or history) presentations sometimes appear to be related to cell position. When, for instance, the theory is general, systematic, dense, drawn from outside a case, and considerable in amount, then the commentary is likely to be extensively discussed before and/or after the case itself, with systematic discussion of "important" events in the case. General theory left more implicit than explicit leads the author merely to present or sum up the overall case, relating it to a body of general theory, rather than discussing it intensively. In monographs, when sizeable cases are introduced, their contribution to the monograph's style is also related to cell position. For instance, a substantive theoretical commentary drawn from outside the research must be introduced to the reader and related to the case: in detail if the theory is systematic and dense, but in far less detail if only bits of a theory are used or are applied without much density. On the other hand, substantive theory which is discovered by the author of a case does not require introduction as such, but is more likely to be woven into the case itself or even into its very construction. Even the stylistic use of very short cases, in monographs or articles, seems partly to reflect the theory's cell position—as when, following stratification theory, an author presents an interview (or interview fragments) from three interviewees arranged by their social class position;[22] or

---

20. *Op. cit.*

21. *The Urban Villagers* (New York: The Free Press of Glencoe, 1962).

22. Lee Rainwater, *Family Design* (Chicago; Aldine Publishing Company, 1965), pp. 73-79.

when numbers of cases are presented serially and each analyzed in turn, as Shibutani did with cases about "rumors" in order to develop an excellent substantive theory about rumor.[23]

There is another reason for emphasizing the relationship of style and type of theoretical commentary. The use of cases or case histories within long case studies probably is more inventive, and certainly more various, than researchers realize. Many researchers incorporate cases—both short and long into their publications without a clear focus on how they do so, since their attention almost invariably is much more on analysis and evidence than on the cases themselves. In a previous publication by one of us (and his co-authors),[24] several different kinds of cases were introduced, in a variety of ways and for a variety of reasons.[25] None of the authors were fully aware —and probably their readers are even less aware—of the range of types, modes, and functions of their cases. Since case histories are so widely used by social scientists, a much closer scrutiny of them is warranted, both by those who publish cases, in any form, and by their readers. Both share the responsibility of course for fuller recognition of how cases are used and for what purposes. Closer scrutiny should lead to increasingly innovative uses and construction of case histories. We hope this further attention might also lead to increasing publication of long case histories—and also to more effective case study monographs.

Another important question—related especially to a case study's style and its type of theoretical commentary—is what kind of *comparative analysis* is offered by the author? When his publication includes two or more cases, then some kind of contrast will be drawn between or among them, either explicitly by the researcher or implicitly by the reader, and usually by both. Even when a case study publication consists of only a single case, (say a riot) its author is very likely to make comments which indicate how this case differs and is similar to other cases; if not, his readers unquestionably, unless they are very uncritical, will draw such contrasts for themselves. Such comparative analyses are not always of the same type or made

---

23. *Op. cit.* One critical reader has remarked, however, that Shibutani's cases sometimes seem directly related to the evidential points he draws from them, but sometimes he merely applies to them a distant —and perhaps "not too pertinent"—theory drawn mainly from Park and Mead.

24. Anselm L. Strauss, Leonard Schatzman, Rue Bucher, Danuta Ehrlich, and Melvin Sabshin, *Psychiatric Ideologies and Instructions* (New York: The Free Press of Glencoe, 1964).

25. Cf. also Anselm L. Strauss, *Images of the American City* (New York: The Free Press of Glencoe, 1961).

for the same purposes. For instance, Gouldner's early study of bureaucratic function in a factory was a one case research, designed to elaborate and correct a theory of bureaucracy derived mainly from Max Weber.[26] In a later study of bureaucracy, Blau gave two constructed cases (work groups in federal agencies).[27] Blau's comparative analysis also served to elaborate and correct a general theory of bureaucracy. A recent study by Crozier contrasts three French governmental agencies, highlighting the differences of their bureaucratic features as well as their similarities because both agencies are French—hence their peculiar differences from non-French types of bureaucracy.[28]

The range of purposes and styles of comparative analyses reflected in the above case *studies* can be better appreciated by contrasting several single case *histories*. Thus Sutherland's case history of the professional thief uses comparative analyses in two principal ways. First, he explicitly comments, mainly in amplifying footnotes, to show how other "con men's" lives and activities are usually similar, but at times dissimilar. Second, Sutherland also makes clear comparisons among different types of professional thieves to distinguish them from con men. Third, he implicitly contrasts their careers and activities with other types of criminals. The analysis is carried out partly in rather descriptive terms and partly in terms of general sociological theory.

On the other hand, the classic life history by Thomas and Znaniecki begins with a three-fold typology of men, and then offers the personal history of a Pole who exemplifies one type. Commenting in footnotes and before and after the case, they make comparisons with other Polish emigants in accordance with the general and substantive theories thoroughly discussed in the preceding four volumes of their five volume work.

In our own commentary on the case history of Mrs. Abel, the other contrasts, with the type of pain and dying trajectories exemplified by her story, are explicitly and repeatedly made, both in general and with regard to specific details of the patient's story. Internal comparisons also are made of various phases of Mrs. Abel's pain and dying trajectories, as well as with corresponding phases in other types of pain and dying careers.

---

26. Alvin W. Gouldner, *Patterns of Industrial Bureaucracy* (New York: The Free Press of Glencoe, 1954) and C .W. Mills and H. Gerth (eds.), *From Max Weber* (New York: Oxford University Press, 1946).

27. Peter Blau, *The Dynamics of Bureaucracy* (Chicago: The University of Chicago Press, 1955).

28. Michel Crozier, *The Bureaucratic Phenomenon* (Chicago: The University of Chicago Press, 1964).

The types of comparative analyses used in the above case studies and histories can be highlighted further by contrasting them with the article by Shellow and Roemer about "The Riot That Didn't Happen" because Shellow and Roemer helped to prevent its occurrence.[29] This non-riot is described as a "case," and the theoretical analysis explicitly contrasts it only with riots that have occurred. The analysis turns around the conditions for riots which were absent because of certain tactics used by the police who were consulting with the researchers.

We are emphasizing the differential styles and the comparative analyses utilized in various case studies and histories for two reasons. First, we wish to advocate a more self-conscious use of these analyses in studies and in commentaries for case histories. Since researchers seem very little aware of their comparative use of cases, elsewhere we have detailed how comparative analyses differ immensely from publication to publication; the same can be said of the case materials on which comparative analyses are made.[30]

Second, and much the more important reason, we wish to advocate that researchers publish from their data *many more* case histories, *selecting* cases in accordance with clearly thought-out comparative analyses. Probably most lone case histories have tended to be selected on the basis of luck in obtaining them or are pulled out of larger bodies of data because they were "fuller" than other cases; while short case histories within monographs and articles are more likely to be presented, or constructed, because they illustrate or give evidence for points that the researcher is attempting to establish. Yet this selection is likely to be deficient if the researcher is not quite clear as to the functioning of his comparative analysis—and in terms which we have used earlier, his conception cannot be quite clear if he does not know how his analysis related to the level, source, systematization of density of his theory. Moreover, his theory should provide the basis for selecting the case histories which when presented will give the best merging of theoretical commentary and case history material.

In conclusion, we hope that sociologists by using this book both as an example and as a starting point will clearly demarcate case histories from case studies and will start doing the former with the came clarity of purpose that now characterizes the latter—the publication of case histories surely has considerable merit as part of the total sociological enterprise.

---

29. Social Problems, Vol. 14 (Fall, 1966).

30. *This Discovery of Grounded Theory, op .cit.,* Chapter 2, pp. 21-45.